OXFORD MEDICAL PUBLICATIONS

Coronary heart disease

THE FACTS

Coronary heart disease

THE FACTS

J. P. SHILLINGFORD

Emeritus Professor of Cardiovascular Medicine,
Royal Postgraduate Medical School, London

OXFORD
OXFORD UNIVERSITY PRESS
NEW YORK TORONTO
1981

Oxford University Press, Walton Street, Oxford OX2 6DP
London Glasgow New York Toronto
Delhi Bombay Calcutta Madras Karachi
Kuala Lumpur Singapore Hong Kong Tokyo
Nairobi Dar Es Salaam Cape Town
Melbourne Wellington

and associate companies in
Beirut Berlin Ibadan Mexico City

Published in the United States
by Oxford University Press, New York

British Library Cataloguing in Publication Data

Shillingford, J P
    Coronary heart disease. – (Oxford
    medical publications).
    1. Coronary heart disease
    I. Title   II. Series
    616.1'23   RC685.C6   80-41458
    ISBN 0-19-261262-X

Typeset by Hope Services, Abingdon
Printed in Great Britain
by R. Clay & Co. Ltd., Bungay

Contents

Introduction

BY A PATIENT WHO IS A UNIVERSITY PROFESSOR

It was an overcast day in early August. I remember it well for other reasons. I had been invited by a senior colleague to his club to meet a foreign visitor. We had lunched elegantly, but not unwisely. Driving there, or it may have been on the way back (I forget), I had had some pain in the chest, and an indefinable sense of malaise which would not be ignored. The pain had gone away, as had some similar pain three weeks before. It was certainly not overpowering, because I remember doing one or two pieces of shopping on the way back. But it had disturbed me, so that before the afternoon was out I had seen a doctor, and before the day was over I had been admitted to hospital. I had had, my doctor said, 'an ischaemic episode'. In spite of this, I surprised the sister on the cardiac ward because I walked in there.

I slept most of the next day and felt greatly refreshed. I spent three weeks, up and about, convalescing. These three weeks passed pleasantly enough, partly in boredom, partly in readjustment, even sometimes in humour, as when I woke one night to find an anxious nurse bending over me because my cardiac monitor, but not my heart, had ceased to function! We were both relieved, she to find me still alive, I to go back to sleep.

However, all this was only the lull before the storm. Three days after returning home, quite abruptly, I felt unwell. Within an hour I was in severe pain and seriously ill. I was admitted to the same ward, but this time not on foot! My progress was stormy, but eventually successful. When the great day came, five weeks later, that I was discharged home once more, it was a beginning rather than an end.

Convalescence was leisurely. It needed to be. It was four months before I was well enough to do any kind of work, six before I was working full time, and twelve before I felt that I was really back to earning my keep. In this time there were ups and downs, good days and bad days. Sooner or later, though, my determination to discard invalidism and to return to normality meant that the trend was inexorably upwards, even if sometimes it was uphill. There were compensations. My son was six at the time. We saw more of each other in these weeks and months than we would otherwise ever have done. Together we read all seven books of C. S. Lewis's *Chronicles of Narnia*, day by day, uninterruptedly over a long period of time. This all took place ten years ago, and the highlight of my rehabilitation was a family holiday in Switzerland. We had three weeks in a chalet in Canton Vaud. I walked in the mountains, spent long hours lying in Alpine pastures reading to my children, and returned to England, to my work and to the *status quo ante*.

And yet it was not quite the *status quo ante*. It was the *status quo* with a plus. There was a new element in my living. I had never been a valetudinarian. I had never been diet-conscious, bowel-conscious, heart-conscious, or, indeed, health-conscious at all. Now, there was something with which I must come to terms. In spite of a major heart attack my exercise tolerance was good. I went back with zest to my garden, and then to the development of the garden of the house to which we moved to be nearer my work. True, I had some residual angina (chest pain on major effort), but this was not troublesome, and it can be avoided with skill, restraint, and the occasional use of trinitrin tablets. I was also prescribed some other tablets, which I take to this day, and which my doctor assures me make my heart work more efficiently.

My aim was to lead an essentially normal life, and this I

have, in large measure, achieved in the ten years since the events I have described. There have been three factors which have contributed to this. In the first place, I have concealed my past wherever possible, though not deceitfully. I have not talked, thought, or lived in the world of illness and doctors any more than has been absolutely necessary. This side of my life has, in other words, been kept in its place. That is was a place it would be foolish to deny. That it was no bigger place than necessary has been my policy. The second factor has been the avoidance of various things which make life more difficult for a healthily functioning but admittedly scarred heart. I have mentioned one already. We moved house so as to give me a relatively short and comparatively easy journey to work by public transport, and so that I did not have a twice daily car journey. I did not cease to drive, but in practice, when there is driving to be done, I usually share it equally with my wife. In everyday life I have learnt to avoid heavy and rushed meals, or committing myself to exercise or a hurried journey immediately after a meal. Late nights are undesirable, although an occasional one is not unmanageable. Disturbed nights are bad. Enforced haste, especially if there is luggage or even a heavy briefcase to cope with, is anathema. Exercise itself is good, especially walking. I do not jog. I unashamedly ask a younger man to help with, or actually do, a piece of heavy lifting. In the winter, I can do anything outdoors provided I am really warmly clad. Cold rooms are to be avoided, especially bedrooms and bathrooms. I do not allow myself to be over-weight. In practice, this is not a very difficult list to cope with, and in any case the principle for recovered coronary patients is to be 'wise as serpents and harmless as doves', and being one step ahead of events and circumstances, by taking thought, is really not a very high price to pay for the avoidance of difficulties.

However, so far I have spoken of negative things. There have been four positive influences and supports. In the first place I should not have been writing this at all if I had not been brought through what, in the argot of medical practice, was euphemistically termed 'an ischaemic episode' with skill and experience by the doctors involved. Equally important, my own particular doctor has been forward-looking and positive-thinking, and has worked, with me, towards a return to normal living within the not very onerous bounds inevitably imposed by the facts. My second good fortune was an understanding and indulgent employer, who waited patiently for my return, and was the soul of unhurried kindness in the early months, allowing me to tailor my work to suit my returning abilities. To both of these I owe an immeasurable debt. However, my strength lay, above all, in having a wife who refused either to be shaken by the seriousness of the situation at the beginning or, later on, to succumb to the temptation to impose upon me a life of invalidism. We both saw to it that I did not become condemned by my illness and its residuum of minor disability to a life apart from others. We have lived on the basis of our life being somewhere on a continuum. At one end is perfect health, at the other severe disability. We have reckoned to live much nearer one end than the other. This merges, perhaps, with the fourth factor, which is that we both see eye to eye in having a spiritual outlook on life which enables us with ease to integrate such episodes, and the continuing situations which ensue, into our scheme of things, and are left neither disturbed nor unsatisfied. After all everyone, even the doctors themselves, must come to terms with this sooner or later.

1

The incidence of coronary heart disease

There can be few people who have not heard of coronary heart disease. The illness is no respecter of persons and may strike presidents of the super-powers or the ordinary man in the street. Primarily a disease of advancing age, it also frequently attacks the middle-aged and, in some cases, the young.

The 'furring up' of our arteries which is the basic cause of coronary heart disease occurs not only in man but under certain conditions is also found in other species of the animal kingdom.

Although coronary heart disease has occurred throughout the ages and was well known to doctors in the eighteenth and nineteenth centuries, the rapid advance in diagnostic methods and improved treatment, together with the publicity given by the media, has made it appear to be on the increase. Some authorities believe that this increase is real and, indeed, coronary heart disease has been called the 'modern epidemic'. The number of people dying of this disease as recorded by the death certificates in Great Britain during 1942 was 18 591. Twenty years later in 1962 the number of deaths recorded had risen to 102 478, more than a five-fold increase. At present the number of deaths annually from cardiovascular disease is more than twice those due to all forms of cancer.

It would seem likely that the increased size of the population and the improved expectancy of life, with the consequent rise in the age of the population, have contributed to the increase, together with more accurate diagnosis and certification of cause of death.

Coronary heart disease accounts for about 80 per cent of all sudden deaths and so the number of recorded sudden deaths can be used as an index of the real or absolute increase in this disease. The Registrar General's *Statistical Review for England and Wales* shows that in 1942 the mortality rate (number of sudden deaths per 1 million persons living) was 105 for males and 103 for females, but by 1962 it had risen to 149 and 151 respectively and continued to rise until recently, when, in the USA in particular, there is evidence that it has begun to fall. The UK figures depend on the awareness of the Coroner's pathologist of the likelihood of thrombosis of the coronary arteries being responsible for sudden death.

Whether or not there has been a real increase in the incidence of the disease, it is without doubt one of the major killers of our century, in spite of the tremendous amount of research, both past and present, that has gone into the nature of the disease and its more effective treatment.

2

How the heart works

It is not possible to understand fully exactly what either a heart attack or coronary arterial disease is without a simple, basic knowledge of how the heart is constructed and how it works. When we consider that, with all our ingenuity, we have not yet been able to devise a pump that will run for up to 100 years without attention, we realize what a remarkable organ the heart is.

The heart consists of four separate pumps which are beautifully controlled in rhythm and sequence by small electric currents which cause the muscular walls of the chambers of the pump to contract and expel blood through the arteries of the body. These chambers bear the Latin names of atria and ventricles, one pair situated approximately on the right side of the heart and the other pair on the left.

Blood from the rest of the body is returned by the veins to the right atrium. The right atrium is a thin-walled sac situated at the upper part of the heart that is capable of contracting by muscular action. The contraction is initiated by a small electric current produced at regular intervals by a collection of cells in the upper part of the atrium known as the sino-atrial node. This can be compared to the ignition system of a motor car which produces an electrical current at regular intervals to fire the sparking plugs. In health, at rest, the electric current is produced at approximately 80 times a minute and is reflected in the rate of the heart beat and the pulse.

The sino-atrial node is under the control of nervous impulses from the brain, so that when we are excited for example, when we are going for an interview, taking an examination or before competitive sport, our pulse may quicken and we may notice the rapid beating of the heart. Conversely under extreme conditions the brain may cause the pulse to slow and produce a fainting attack; this is well illustrated by the effect of the sight of blood or surgical operations on some people. The sino-atrial node, or 'pace-maker', as it is sometimes called, can also respond in rate to the amount of blood returning to the heart and thus indirectly control the heart's output of blood.

The right atrium opens into a second chamber with a thick muscular wall, known as the right ventricle. Between these two chambers there is the tricuspid valve, which is made up of three slips of thin tissue fixed at their periphery to the opening between the atrium and ventricle and anchored at their free edges to the muscular part of the ventricle by string-like cords. The whole mechanism acts as a one-way valve allowing blood to pass from the atrium into the ventricle but not to be returned when the ventricle contracts.

The right ventricle is responsible for pumping blood into the lungs and contracts rhythmically after the right atrium so that the blood is passed sequentially from the atrium into the ventricle. The atrium contracts when the ventricle is relaxed and has its maximum potential capacity. The ventricle then contracts, the tricuspid valve closes, and the blood is expelled into the blood vessels of the lungs. Between the right ventricle and the arteries of the lungs is another valve made up of three leaflets (the pulmonary valve) which prevent the blood passing backwards into the ventricle from the lungs.

The main artery to the lungs divides into two main branches, one to the right, and one to the left lung. The main arteries further break up into a myriad of small branches similar to the branches of a tree with its numerous twigs and by this means blood is carried to the numerous air sacs of the lungs where it picks up oxygen and loses carbon dioxide during the process of breathing.

The blood, now full of oxygen, is collected up by the veins

How the heart works

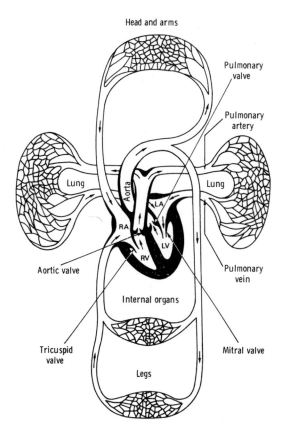

Fig. 1. Diagrammatic representation of the circulation of the blood from the heart (see text).

of the lungs and returned to the left side of the heart via four main veins to the left atrium, similar in structure to the right atrium. The right and left atria are separated by a fibro-muscular wall. The left atrium drains into the left ventricle through a large opening guarded by another valve known as the mitral valve and the mechanism of filling of the left ventricle is similar to that of the right.

The left ventricle is the main pump of the heart responsible for pumping blood right through the body at the rate of about a gallon a minute at rest, rising to up to four gallons on exercise and maintaining a maximum pressure of up to 150 millimetres of mercury in health. Blood is expelled from the left ventricle into the main artery of the body (the aorta). Once again the blood is only allowed in a one-way direction by a three leaflet valve (aortic valve) at the junction of the left ventricle and aorta.

When the ventricle contracts the valve opens and blood is expelled into the aorta. When the ventricle relaxes the pressure in the aorta is higher than in the ventricle and the valve snaps shut producing a sound that can be heart through a stethoscope placed on the surface of the chest.

The natural rhythm and orderly sequence of the heart beat is controlled by electrical connections through specialized muscle fibres from the sino-atrial node throughout the whole heart by a specialized network of tissues passing from the atria to the ventricles.

The blood supply of the heart itself (see Plate 1), the coronary arterial system, begins from two openings in the wall of the aorta or main vessel leaving the heart. One of the major coronary arteries extends over the right and back sides of the ventricular muscle mass and is called the right coronary artery. The other artery supplies chiefly the left side, part of the front and the back of the heart muscle and is known as the left coronary artery. These two major coronary arteries are responsible for almost all of the blood that is available for the heart muscle. The left coronary artery soon branches into two major divisions, one supplying the front of the left ventricular muscle and the other the back of the heart. As in the case of arteries elsewhere throughout the body, they break up into many smaller arteries to supply individual muscle fibres throughout the whole heart. It is of great importance that some of these small arteries inter-connect with each other so that, if the blood supply diminishes through one major artery, the other is able to take over through these small junctions, which are known as anastomoses, and protect the heart from damage from lack of oxygen and nutrients.

3

Changes in the coronary arteries and blood leading to a heart attack

Atherosclerosis

Atherosclerosis is the process in which the lining (endo-thelium) of the arteries thickens with the deposition of fatty substances and cholesterol. The thickened areas are usually found in patches which vary greatly in size. To a greater or lesser degree this process is going on in all of us. It increases with advancing age, and is associated with 'hardening of the arteries'. The cause of this change is unknown but family history, high blood-pressure, obesity, and smoking may play a part in accelerating the development of atherosclerosis.

In the coronary arteries the thickenings often involve the whole circumference of the structure and can cause all degrees of narrowing from quite a minor amount down to complete occlusion and obstruction of the blood passing through the artery.

When the diseased part of the artery is examined under the

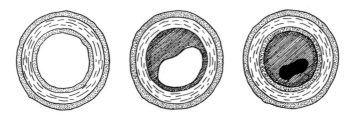

Fig. 2. The development of atheriosclerosis (or 'furring up' of the arteries). *Left:* a normal artery; *centre:* a narrowed artery; *right:* a blood clot completely blocking the artery.

11

microscope it is seen to be composed of an accumulation of fat and cholesterol surrounded by a scar. In places, the surrounding tissue dies and forms an ulcerating patch on the surface of the lining of the artery. Calcium (chalk) may be deposited and further stiffen and harden the artery into a rigid, narrowed, tube.

Thrombosis

The blood is made up of red and white cells together with smaller cells known as platelets, all suspended in the fluid called plasma which carries nutrients and chemicals round the circulation. Normally the blood is fluid and flows freely. When it comes into contact with an injured surface as, for example, a cut in a finger, complex changes occur so that the platelets and other cells adhere together with the production of protein named fibrin, and produce a clot. This is nature's way of preventing further bleeding.

The process of clot or 'thrombus' formation may occur within the arteries themselves if the lining is damaged by atherosclerosis and ulceration. When the blood and especially the platelets are stimulated by a break in the arterial lining they are attracted to the defect and put out small projections which adhere to each other and form a plug. At the same time they liberate a number of chemicals which cause the artery to contract.

Although clotting is a vital process in the preventing of haemorrhage, it may produce harmful and unwanted effects in the coronary arteries. The formation of a clot produced by the accumulation of platelets may cause the artery to contract (spasm) leading to anginal pain, or block it altogether, leading to a heart attack (coronary thrombosis). Small pieces of the platelet 'thrombus' may break off and lodge in smaller branches of the coronary artery causing further pain. Much research work has been put into developing drugs to diminish the likelihood of the platelets adhering to each other within the coronary arteries without having undesirable side-effects. These compounds are discussed later in this book (Chapter 8).

Clot or thrombus formation in the arteries is a different process from that in the veins or in the chambers of the heart. Another group of medicines known as the anti-coagulants (coumarin, warfarin) are effective under the latter conditions, but do not appear to be of value in preventing the formation of thrombi in the coronary arteries. These medicines are given when there is evidence of serious thrombosis in the veins of the legs or there is an irregularity of heart action which may lead to the formation of clots within the heart itself.

4

Risk factors and prevention

Over the last few years a great deal of research and very large sums of money have been spent to discover whether it is possible to alter the incidence of heart disease by altering people's life-style. At the same time, the life-styles of different populations have been studied in relation to their incidence of coronary heart disesase. Unfortunately, it takes a long period of time for the results of such research to become apparent. Coronary heart disease is a slow, progressive condition which may develop over a patient's whole lifetime and the results of alterations in diet, exercise, living conditions, or drugs may not be seen until many years later.

It is of considerable interest, however, that research has clearly shown that there are important differences in the fre-

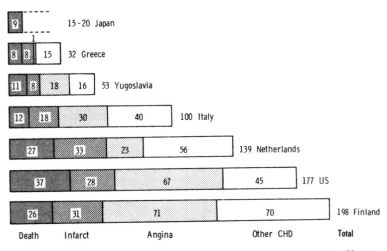

Fig. 3. The relative incidence of coronary heart disease in different countries (incidence rates per 10 000 men aged 40–59).

quency of coronary heart disease in different countries and within different population groups. In some countries there is a high incidence among young adults and middle-aged persons, while in others heart disease is rare in these groups. It is on these facts that many of the measures suggested for preventing the disease have been based. Figure 3 shows the incidence of coronary heart disease for men between the ages of 40 and 59 years in various countries in the world. This has been divided into death, actual heart attacks, and angina and it will be seen that in Japan the incidence of the disease is negligable, whereas in Finland it is high. It has been suggested that diet is responsible for these differences; in the West our usual diet is high in saturated fat, cholesterol, and calories with the result that there is a high level of fats and cholesterol in the blood. The habit of cigarette smoking and a raised blood pressure are additional so-called risk factors in the development of the disease. There would also appear to be a familial tendency; the disease often runs in families. It is difficult to separate out whether this is due to an inherited characteristic or whether these families share a similar diet together with the other risk factors, such as smoking.

The so-called risk factors must, therefore, include family history, smoking, high blood fats, and high blood pressure. Many other factors have been suggested at various times, including hard and soft water, insufficient fibre in the diet, stress, personality, and excessive consumption of sugar, but, so far, not one of them has been found in itself to be a primary factor in the incidence of heart disease.

Family history

Recent careful work has been carried out in East Finland where the incidence of coronary heart disease is very high. The occurrence of the main coronary risk factors was assessed in the families of 211 men under the age of 56 years from East Finland. Fifty were survivors of a recent heart attack, 55 had died of the attack, and 53 suffered from angina. Another 53 were healthy men used for comparison or reference. Familial high blood fat was found to be twice as common and familial high blood pressure three times as common in patients suffering with coronary heart disease as those who were used as the reference patients and who were free from all evidence of the disease. It would appear, therefore, from this work that there are familial traits in the development of coronary disease and the most impressive correlation appears to be with a maternal history of the illness.

It should be emphasized, however, that many people develop heart disease without any family history at all, while others, with a family history, may lead long lives free from the disease. All one can say is that it is somewhat more likely that one will develop coronary heart disease if there is a significant family history.

Cigarette smoking

The consumption of manufactured cigarettes has vastly increased in each decade of this century and, increasingly, younger people and women are beginning to smoke. The evidence for the role of cigarette smoking in coronary heart disease comes from a large number of studies of the population. These almost conclusively indicate a strong association between the habit of cigarette smoking and the subsequent development of coronary artery disease. Overall there is about a 70 per cent greater chance of developing coronary disease among average cigarette smokers than non-smokers. However, the frequency among younger smokers is many times higher than among non-smokers of the same age. (The mortality risk from all causes is also greater for smokers of both sexes and all ages. Almost 80 per cent of the excess mortality can be explained by diseases that are related to smoking.)

The risk of coronary heart disease increases according to the number of cigarettes smoked, the duration of the smoking habit, the age of starting smoking, and the amount of smoke inhaled. The greatest relative excess risk of coronary heart disease is among younger subjects smoking 40 or more cigarettes a day. The evidence is not so clear for the role, if any, of any other forms of smoking, and it would appear that pipe smoking is not such a serious risk, mainly perhaps because the smoke is not inhaled as is cigarette smoke. Heavy smoking of cigars probably carries a risk similar to that of smoking cigarettes. We do not yet know which factors in cigarette smoke produce the increased incidence of coronary heart disease, but examination of the umbilical arteries of babies born to mothers who smoke very heavily shows them to be narrowed (see also Chapter 6, p. 30). Smoking may also accentuate other risk factors.

In summary, therefore, one of the risk factors that has been shown to be amenable to alteration is that of smoking, especially in the young, so giving up smoking will certainly lessen the chance of having a heart attack.

Dietary fats and cholesterol

Although it has been conclusively shown that a high blood cholesterol is associated with a higher incidence of coronary heart disease, not all doctors agree that a strict diet initiated in middle age will favourably affect one's chances of developing the disease. Much more research has to be done to establish firmly that there is a relationship between the fats in the diet and the incidence of coronary heart disease.

People manufacture their own cholesterol in the liver and there is a wide variation from person to person, not only in the amount of cholesterol they manufacture from other substances but also in the absorption of cholesterol and fats from the diet and the way in which they are used in the body; it may well be that genetic factors are important in this variation.

Moreover, the composition of fats is very complicated and each fat can be split into a number of components. It has recently been found that some of these components are actually protective as far as the development of atheroma in the arteries is concerned. Included in the composition of the fats circulating in the blood are so-called high-density lipoproteins (HDL), low-density lipoproteins (LDL), and very low density lipoproteins (VLDL). It would appear that the HDL component is protective against the production of atheroma, whereas the LDL and VLDL fractions increase the risk of its development. There are also other components known as fatty acids, some of which are protective against blood clotting.

It will be seen, therefore, that the whole subject of fats and the development of coronary heart disease is far from clear and there is still considerable controversy among cardiologists and scientists about the relative advantages of changing our normal diet, and further research is needed. Perhaps all we can safely say is that, whatever your age, it will do no harm to reduce intake of all fats, and to substitute margarine and vegetable cooking oils (polyunsaturated fats) for animal fats (saturated fats).

Carbohydrates

Another common controversy about diet is concerned with carbohydrates. Some authorities believe that an excessive intake of carbohydrates produces a higher concentration of fat in the blood. But, to set against this theory, is the observation that the Japanese, who eat a lot of carbohydrates, do not have high blood fats by Western standards.

There is no firm evidence from either laboratory experimental observations or population epidemiological evidence that carbohydrate intake is directly the cause of coronary heart disease. It must be remembered, however, that excessive carbohydrate intake leads to obesity, which, in itself, is a risk factor in the development of high blood pressure.

Dietary fibre

It has been suggested that lack of fibre in the form of vegetables, nuts, and whole bran is the source of many of the ills of Western man, from bowel disturbances to heart disease. The analysis of 'fibre' is extremely difficult, as there are many chemical types which appear to have different actions on the body's function and absorption from the bowel. Many give bulk to the food as it passes through the bowels and may modify the absorption of cholesterol and other fats. Although the consumption of fibre such as bran and bran products may be useful in preventing constipation there is still controversy as to whether they play a significant part in the development of coronary heart disease.

Perhaps the best advice that can be given on diet generally is not to eat more than is necessary to maintain a lean body weight (reducing the intake of animal fats can do no harm), keep to the golden rule of 'moderation in all things', and, in view of the present uncertainty of the role of food in the production of coronary disease, do not become a food faddist or even neurotic over what you eat.

High blood pressure

There is strong evidence that a raised blood pressure is related to the risk of developing coronary heart disease. What is not so clear is whether treating raised blood pressure once it is established reduces the incidence of coronary attacks. Research is under way in several countries to try and determine the exact relationship between treated and untreated patients, and their subsequent development of coronary disease.

Coronary heart disease: the facts

Exercise

Exercise, or lack of it, is a subject of considerable controversy as a 'risk factor'. Much work has been carried out to see whether physical activity is related to the development of coronary heart disease and, although there may be a positive protective effect of regular physical activity, it is extremely difficult to eliminate bias and assess the total activity, both at leisure and work, of a group of people. Not a few of the world's leading marathon runners have developed coronary artery disease, and the hard-working lumberjacks of East Finland have a very high incidence of the illness.

However, moderate, pleasurable exercise improves the general muscular fitness of the body and leads to general wellbeing and a greater enjoyment of life; for this reason alone, exercise is to be recommended even if there is no strong evidence that in itself it will prevent a heart attack. Violent exercise such as squash and competitive running is best avoided after middle age, as sudden death has been recorded in these circumstances.

'Stress'

Most people consider that 'stress' or a person's response to stress may have something to do with the development of heart attacks and this has led to the claim by some doctors in the United States that people can be divided into type A and type B personalities. Type A personalities, with a sense of aggression and urgency and with a continuous struggle within themselves and with society; said to be more likely to have coronary disease. There are, however, very many type A people who never develop coronary disease and vice versa. In practice it is very difficult to change someone's personality in order to reduce the associated risk that this involves, and the stress theory remains interesting but difficult, if not impossible, to prove with certainty.

Risk factors and prevention

Can we prevent a heart attack?

Although the incidence of coronary disease appeared to rise dramatically and relentlessly in the United States over the period 1940–68 there has been a fall of over 20 per cent in the eight-year period from 1968–76. This change has prompted many research workers to look for underlying causes and to see whether the incidence can be reduced even further in the future.

The changes in diet have been extensively studied. The consumption of vegetable fat tripled between 1909 and 1973, while there was only a modest increase in that of animal fat. This move has resulted in a lower average blood cholesterol in the population as a whole. The consumption of linoleic acid, which may play a part in the regulation of thrombosis, has increased along with the consumption of polyunsaturated fats.

There is controversy as to whether the small fall in the blood cholesterol could affect the incidence of the disease and this factor has to be separated from the other changes in the life habits of people in the United States.

Data from one study in Framingham, Massachusetts, USA show that between 1950 and 1968 the prevalence of ciga-rette smokers declined from 61 per cent to 37 per cent in men and from 40 per cent to 31 per cent among women. Surveys among large populations carried out by the national Clearing House for Smoking and Health confirmed a decline in the percentage of male smokers in every decade from 21 to 65 years and older, between 1964 and 1975. The percentage of male cigarette smokers declined from 53 per cent to 37 per cent and female from 32 per cent to 29 per cent.

During the last few years there has been an explosive increase in interest in outdoor and leisure activities involving exercise of which the much-publicized habit of jogging is only the tip of the iceberg. Although it cannot be proved, this change from a sedentary life to physical activity, if real

Coronary heart disease: the facts

(many children and adults still remain sitting in front of television sets), may have played a part in the change in the development of the disease.

There was no effective treatment for high blood pressure until the 1950s. Since then the introduction of specific medicines has allowed us to control high blood pressure in an ever-increasing number of people, and this has brought about an improvement in mortality from cardiovascular disease as a whole.

No other detectable changes such as stress, change in family history, alterations in water hardness, or other suggested agents causing coronary disease have been proved to have taken place over the period in which the incidence of coronary heart disease fell.

It must be emphasized that these results are obtained on the population as a whole and no allowance made for individual susceptibilities. The main message that appears to come out of these observations is that, if you wish to lower the risk of an attack, stop smoking cigarettes, eat sparingly and perhaps reduce animal fats, have your blood pressure checked at yearly intervals over the age of 50, and take moderate, and preferably pleasurable, exercise.

If you take these precautions the risk of a heart attack will be lowered but in spite of them you may still develop the disease. As far as possible life should be lived to the full and excessive concern over what may happen if you eat certain foods or have not taken daily exercise cannot but spoil its enjoyment.

5

Diagnosis

Although a history of pain in the chest associated with exercise, emotion, or heavy meals is likely to be associated with coronary artery disease, further tests have to be performed before a definitive diagnosis can be made.

The electrocardiogram

The most valuable of all these tests is the electrocardiogram (ECG) and the final diagnosis cannot be safely made without its use. The electrocardiograph is an instrument which picks up the very small electrical signals generated by the heart from the surface of the body, amplifies them, and records them either on an oscilloscope (rather like a television screen) or on a paper chart. The electrical impulses can be detected from various areas of the heart by placing electrodes over different parts of the body. Those placed on the arms record the electrical activity in the front part of the heart and those on the legs and arms on the underside and back of the heart. More accurate estimations are made by placing further electrodes across the front of the chest. Normally twelve such records are made and this is known as the standard 12-lead electrocardiogram.

The electrocardiogram can not only show whether or not the patient has angina due to coronary heart disease but also whether there are any irregularities of rhythm within the heart. The interpretation of the record needs considerable experience and sometimes the services of a specialist. The procedure of taking the record is quite painless and the patient does not feel any discomfort at all.

In some cases of angina the record taken with the patient

at rest may be perfectly normal, and it is only when the patient exercises and produces the pain of angina that the electrical record becomes abnormal by showing up the areas of the heart which are becoming relatively starved of blood on exercise. An exercise test is made by either asking the patient to walk up and down a few steps, to ride a fixed bicycle, or to walk on a treadmill. All these methods of exercising have the same result—namely, to increase the work of the heart.

The electrocardiogram is a definitive method of confirming the presence of coronary heart disease in most cases. In some instances, however, the electrocardiogram will give negative results even in the presence of coronary heart disease and further tests may be necessary.

Angiography

Where surgery of the coronary arteries is under consideration it becomes essential to see the outline of the arteries and how much they have been affected by disease. The arteries can be seen in outline only when a radio-opaque substance is passing through them. This is achieved in practice by injecting directly into the coronary arteries, a specialized procedure which is carried out at centres equipped with advanced X-ray apparatus.

Angiography is carried out with the patient lying on the X-ray couch throughout. A small area, either over the artery in the groin or in the arm, is injected with a local anaesthetic. A fine flexible tube (catheter) is passed into the artery and passed into the orifice of one of the coronary arteries. Its passage can be watched on the television screen attached to the X-ray tube and all the procedures recorded on ciné film or video tape. The radio-opaque dye is then injected into the artery and its passage recorded. Each coronary artery is injected in turn and pictures taken with the patient in various positions as the X-ray couch is rotated.

Diagnosis

The records can then be played over and studied at leisure by the radiologist, physician, and surgeon to see whether the narrowed arteries are suitable for repairing or grafting and which parts have to be treated.

Although angiography is for the most part performed in the case of patients who are candidates for coronary artery surgery, it is also of value where the diagnosis is uncertain by other methods and where it is crucial to know the answer, as in the case of airline pilots where the correct diagnosis in doubtful cases of chest pain is vital.

Radio-isotopes

When the heart muscle is damaged by having its blood supply cut off by a coronary artery occlusion it can no longer take up the normal nutrients and chemicals necessary for the maintenance of its action. It has been found possible to use radioactive 'tracer' elements which when injected into the circulation are taken up by the normal but not by the injured muscle. A special camera (gamma camera) placed in front of the chest can detect the radiation produced in the heart and show the damaged area of the heart muscle as a 'cold' spot which appears lighter on the camera's film. The radio-isotope usually used is thallium-201. Not only does this method allow the muscle itself to be visualized, but it also outlines the size of the cardiac chambers and gives an indication of the function of the heart as a whole.

This test can only be performed in specialized heart centres that have the necessary expensive and advanced equipment.

The chest X-ray

The simple X-ray of the chest has a very limited value in showing coronary disease in its early stages. Occasionally calcium may be seen in the coronary arteries. In the later and more serious cases it can show whether the heart is enlarged or whether the lungs are also congested.

Blood tests

In angina there are usually no changes in the blood but it is usually examined to see whether there is anaemia present, as this in itself can lead to or exacerbate angina, or if there are abnormal blood fats. If there has been a heart attack there are several detectable abnormalities and these are described in the section on the coronary care unit.

Ultrasound

When high-frequency sound waves are projected through a fluid they are reflected by any solid structures and the position and depth of those structures from the recording instrument determined. This is the principle behind the depth-finder used at sea, which not only gives the depth of the sea bed but also can detect shoals of fish.

In recent years this principle has been applied to patients to determine the shape of structures underlying the skin.

Ultrasound has a limited application in the diagnosis of coronary disease but is useful in the diagnosis of some of the complications of a heart attack including damaged valves, fluid round the heart, and holes in the heart and can give an indication of how well the heart is performing by measuring how much blood is being expelled at each beat.

26

6

Angina and its treatment

It is possible to have advanced coronary arterial disease without any symptoms at all, providing that sufficient blood flows through the obstructed arteries to reach the heart muscle. When, however, the occlusion reaches approximately 70 per cent of the normal area of the lumen of the arteries the blood supply to the muscle is impaired and it is at this stage that symptoms first appear.

The main symptom is that of pain, often associated with exercise, and known as angina. The term 'angina' comes from the world *angere*, which means to strangle or to suffocate, and was used by William Heberden, a famous physician of the eighteenth century who first gave the classical description of the disease.

The pain of angina, due to a failure of sufficient blood reaching the heart muscle, is usually felt in the front of the chest and may extend all over the chest wall. At times it may move up to the neck and be felt in the jaws or may pass down into the arms and hands, usually on the left side. It may be felt as a heaviness in the wrists or the hands themselves. Occasionally it moves into the back. There is often a sensation of pressure, heaviness, tightness, or constriction of the chest and this may be thought to be due to severe indigestion or 'heartburn'. The type of pain may range from an unpleasant feeling through to an excruciating sensation, associated with sweating or even fear of impending death. Angina is not usually associated with a sharp stabbing or pricking pain which may be knife-like, shooting, burning, cutting, or sharp.

Classically, the pain of angina is brought on by physical effort, emotion, particularly frustration, anxiety or anger, extremes of temperature, especially cold weather, and often after eating a large meal or heavy smoking. It may first make itself apparent when walking fast or uphill and one of its major characteristics is that it goes away on resting. It may only last a few seconds or minutes after which exercise may be resumed.

Patients with angina often have to stop at regular intervals when walking in the street and look in shop windows to rest and relieve themselves of the discomfort. Some patients first notice the symptoms of pain on going out early in the morning into the cold, especially when they are hurrying to catch a train. Pain in the chest associated with any form of exercise, especially if it is relieved by rest, is highly suggestive of angina and medical help in these circumstances should always be sought. The pain of angina is characteristic and quite different from the vague aches and pains that a number of people may have and who suspect that they have heart disease.

In highly strung people any form of emotion, frustration, or anger may cause the heart to beat harder and use more oxygen; in other cases it may cause the coronary arteries to constrict. Anger and frustrations produced at committee meetings have been a not-infrequent source of the development of angina in those susceptible to the illness. Even the excitement associated with watching a boxing fight on television has been the cause of anginal pain.

Anginal pain associated with a heavy meal is more difficult to separate from the pain caused by indigestion and is often thought to be due to the latter. However, those who get anginal pain after eating usually also develop chest pain either on exertion, excitement, or heavy smoking, quite apart from eating.

Although anginal pain is by far the most usual early symptom of coronary disease, narrowing of the coronary artery may cause an irregularity in the heart beat and the first symptom may be a fluttering in the chest, a very slow heart rate, and dizziness or unconsciousness associated with failure of the heart to pump sufficient blood to the brain. Occassionally the action of the heart over a long period may be slowly impaired by an insufficient blood supply due to coronary artery disease but without producing pain. Such patients, especially elderly, may notice the onset of breathlessness and exhaustion. Breathlessness does not mean for certain that one has heart disease, as there are many other causes for this.

Treatment of angina

Remarkable advances have been made in the last few years in both the medical and surgical treatment of angina and much research is at present directed to improving the ways in which the patient may be helped.

Angina is often a most unpleasant symptom and may severely restrict the patient's activities. On the other hand, many patients with angina live long lives and the pain can be well controlled so they can go about their work and normal activities without too much inconvenience.

The cause of the anginal pain is that insufficient blood is reaching the muscle of the heart. This is due to either the 'furring up' of the artery supplying the heart, or to arterial constriction, or a combination of both. The treatment of angina is directed to decreasing the work-load of the heart on the one hand and relieving any coronary artery constriction on the other.

The work-load on the heart and constriction of the coronary arteries can be to some extent controlled by general measures such as attention to smoking, obesity, excessive exercise, excitement, and emotional strain as well as by medicines. In some cases narrowed or blocked arteries can be replaced at surgical operations.

Coronary heart disease: the facts

Smoking

There is clear scientific evidence that smoking not only affects the lungs but also the heart and its blood-vessels. Smoking a cigarette increases the pulse rate and the output of the heart as well as raising the blood pressure. All these three throw an extra load on its reserves. At the same time, smoking has been found to damage the lining of the blood-vessels of the heart in a way which speeds up the 'furring up' process and, indeed, heavy smokers can put their lives in jeopardy if they continue smoking after a heart attack. More recent evidence also suggests that smoking may prevent the manufacture of certain chemicals which in themselves are protecting against thrombosis within the arteries. In some cases smoking itself, possibly because of coronary artery constriction, may provoke an attack of angina, and considerably alter the electrocardiogram when it is taken at the same time as smoking a cigarette.

Experience has shown that it is exceedingly difficult for an habitual smoker to give up the habit, and all the doctor can usually do is to emphasize the harm that is associated with the habit. A pamphlet giving advice can be obtained from the British Heart Foundation, 57 Gloucester Place, London W1H 4DN.

Obesity

Insurance companies have long realized that excessive obesity shortens life and as a result they have loaded premiums for those people who are excessively fat. Excessive weight throws an extra load on the heart, especially on exercise or on walking up stairs. Losing weight for some is almost as difficult as giving up cigarette smoking but in this considerable help may be given by the family or by organizations such as 'Weight Watchers'. One method that may be effective is to have only half the amount of the usual food on one's plate at mealtimes and to avoid eating between meals. To a large extent the amount one eats is a habit and for those who say that they only eat a very small amount yet remain fat it may perhaps be relevant to reflect that nobody in a concentration camp was ever obese. The relation of food to heart disease will be considered in more detail elsewhere (Chapter 14).

Exercise

The pain associated with angina may be looked upon as nature's way of saying that the heart is working too hard and that the patient should slow up as a result. Gentle exercise, therefore—short of producing the pain—will be beneficial but patients who at any time have had any established coronary heart disease should avoid more violent exercise such as hard tennis or squash or jogging. In fact, it is probably good advice to say that anybody over middle-age who is not used to taking very active exercise should avoid it. The incidence of sudden death associated with unaccustomed and more violent forms of exercise in the middle-aged and older is well established.

If you have angina associated with exercise you should walk at a slower pace, avoiding hills and unnecessary stairs if so doing brings on the pain, especially after meals, in the cold, or during periods of emotional stress. Cold is a particularly important precipitating factor and the onset of angina may occur, for example, when you open the front door on a cold morning to walk to work.

The work-load on the heart can be reduced by carefully planning the day's work. For example, arrange to arrive for the train with time to spare and rearrange business and social engagements with reasonable time between them so that unnecessary flurries of physical and mental stress will not occur. Heavy meals also throw an extra load on the heart by the increased blood flow to the stomach and should be avoided, especially if they are followed by exercise and going into the cold. Exercise associated with strenuous static work such as pushing a car which will not start or lifting very heavy loads should definitely be avoided.

Stress

If you are liable to angina and are subject to emotional stress either at work or in the home you should seriously think about readjusting your life to avoid this as much as possible. An excessive mental work-load, irritation with your colleagues, undue ambition, or stress in the home can all lead to the onset of angina.

Drug treatment

Nitrates

One of the mainstays of the treatment of angina over the last hundred years has been a group of drugs known as the nitrates. Of these, glyceryl trinitrate, is the most common. It is usually taken during the acute attack, but may also prevent an attack when taken just before the activity that usually causes one. The action of this drug is to relax the arteries of the whole body including those supplying blood to the heart. In this way the relative blood flow to the heart is increased and the angina relieved.

The usual method of administering this medicine is to prescribe it in the form of tablets which are sucked under the tongue and produce their effect in two or three minutes; the effect lasts up to thirty minutes. Some patients, who are particularly sensitive to the medicine, may find that it gives them a brief but unpleasant headache, flushing, or dizziness. In these circumstances half a tablet may be sucked or a larger one may be spat out immediately its action is felt. This is a relatively harmless remedy and a large number of tablets—

up to twenty a day—may be safely taken. Unfortunately, it is not possible to make the drug in a really effective, long-acting form, although there are several preparations which have variable results and which are taken regularly three or four times a day. Sorbide nitrate takes about five minutes to become effective and lasts up to two hours. Pentaerythritol tetranitrate is a tablet which is swallowed and has a longer, but usually less effective, action than those sucked under the tongue.

Another method of administering the nitrates or nitroglycerine is by an ointment, which is normally applied over a small area of the skin and covered by plaster. This has a longer duration of action than that given under the tongue and is often valuable used at bedtime to prevent pain that comes on at night.

There is no convincing evidence that the nitrates prolong life but, in many instances, they are most effective in removing or reducing the pain associated with angina, and if you are liable to suffer such attacks you should always carry these tablets with you.

Beta blockers

In recent years a whole new series of medicines have been introduced which are known as the beta-blocking agents. The effect of these is to reduce the action of the sympathetic nerve fibres to the heart and blood-vessels, which are involved in emotion, and to regulate the heart rate and force of contraction.

The first of these to be widely used was propranolol (Inderal), which has been found to be highly effective in many patients suffering from angina. Since the introduction of propranolol many other manufacturers have produced beta-blocking agents which have a similar effect (Sotalol, Metropolol, Timolol, Acebutolol, Oxyprenolol, Atenolol, Pindolol). It is only by trial and error that the doctor is able to find out which one is most suitable for any particular patient.

Coronary heart disease: the facts

Propranolol is usually given in divided doses, three times a day, and the dose is so regulated that the normal resting heart-rate is reduced to between 60 and 64 beats a minute. This means that the heart is doing less work than normally. Sometimes when the medicine is first administered there may be a sensation of tiredness and heaviness in the legs and some sleepiness but experience has shown that this wears off in the course of the next week or so and then the side-reactions are very few. In some patients changing to a different formula may alleviate side-effects. It is essential, however, that this medicine be used continuously, as it is only palliative in nature and does not effect a complete cure other than relieving the symptoms of pain.

More recently, some of the pharmaceutical manufacturers have produced beta blockers in long-acting form, e.g. long-acting oxyprendol or propranolol, so that tablets may be taken in the morning and will continue their action throughout the day; this is more convenient than having to remember to take the tablets three or four times a day.

The beta-blocking medicines also have the advantage that they help to control any associated high blood pressure. There is some evidence that their use also prolongs life and may prevent a more serious heart attack.

Calcium antagonists

Another new group of medicines, recently introduced for the control of angina, are known as the calcium antagonists. (Nifedipine). These act by relaxing the arteries and are usually used in association with the beta-blocking medicines if the former on their own are not sufficiently effective.

With the treatment outlined above about 70 per cent of patients are relieved of their symptoms and can lead a normal active life with the minimum of restriction. However, 30 per cent may not gain enough relief or dislike the nuisance of having to take pills continuously. Heart surgery may offer them help and is described elsewhere (Chapter 13).

7

Common questions and answers about angina

Does angina mean I have heart trouble?

Although angina may occasionally be due to other causes such as anaemia, in the majority of cases it is due to coronary artery narrowing, associated with atherosclerosis, which causes the heart pain.

Will it shorten my life?

The outlook for patients with angina is extremely variable and it is never possible to predict, with any accuracy, the effect on longevity. Many patients live many years with angina. Insurance companies, however, will normally 'load' policies where there is a history of the condition.

Will I always have to take tablets?

In a few patients angina improves of its own accord over a period of months or years. In most some form of medication is usually necessary.

Would surgery help?

Heart surgery (coronary artery bypass grafting) relieves the pain in about three-quarters of the patients. This has to be balanced against the severity of the pain, effectiveness of medical treatment, and risk of the operation together with the after-effects of the surgery itself. Judgement as to whether a patient is suitable for heart surgery has to be left to the doctor after a number of special tests have been made.

Is there anything that I can do apart from medicines and surgery?

Giving up smoking and losing weight if you are obese are often helpful. Try to organize your life to avoid those things that bring on the pain; leave plenty of time to catch buses or trains and generally reorganize your life to avoid annoyances.

Should I change my diet?

Beyond keeping slim there is little to worry about altering the diet. Some doctors believe that animal fats should be avoided. It is better to always have small helpings of food and under- rather than over-eat.

Can I drive a car?

Provided that driving does not bring on angina or dizziness it is usually permissible to drive. The licensing authority must be informed of your condition.

Can I fly?

Normally there is no contraindication to flying. The more rarefied air in the aircraft cabin may bring on angina in the occasional patient. The airline can provide oxygen to compensate for the altitude and, if informed ahead, can make arrangements for this to be available if necessary. In most cases a tablet of trinitrin alone will relieve the pain.

How many trinitrin tablets can I take?

The effect of the tablets is very short-lived and up to twenty a day can be safely taken if necessary.

Should I take the trinitrin tablets only if I have the pain?

It is helpful to take such a tablet if you are going to do anything which is known to provoke the pain, such as going into the cold or before sexual intercourse.

Should the 'beta blocking' (e.g. Inderal) tablets make me feel tired and cold?

In some patients there may be a sensation of tiredness and heaviness of the legs, while in others the hands and feet feel cold. This usually wears off in time.

8

Treatment of the coronary attack

Immediate first aid

The coronary attack may come on without warning at any time of day and in any place. Often it may happen in the middle of the night and not only strikes fear in the mind of the patient but in all around him. It is not always clear at which point medical help should be summoned, how this should be done, and what should be done to the patient before help arrives.

The following guide lines should be followed.

1 If the patient complains of very severe pain in the chest which is unbearable and often associated with sweating, nausea, and vomiting, and has lasted for more than half an hour, call your doctor. If he is not readily available ring the ambulance service (999).

2 Before medical help arrives lie the patient flat and if he feels faint raise the legs by placing them on several cushions or a chair.

3 If the patient becomes unconscious and breathing has stopped give two or three sharp blows to the centre of his chest with the clenched fist. If there are two people available one can telephone for the ambulance and the other start mouth-to-mouth respiration and external cardiac massage. (Many members of the public are now being trained in this procedure by organizations including the British Red Cross and St. John's Ambulance Brigade.) If only one person is present call for the ambulance first before performing artificial respiration and compression of the chest as, although the patient can be kept alive by this method, the heart has to be restored to its regular rhythm by means of an electric shock when he reaches hospital.

4 If the pain passes off within half an hour the patient should be kept quietly in bed and the doctor called at the earliest convenient time.

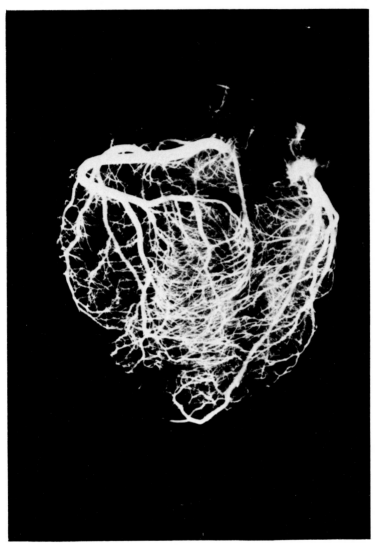

Plate 1. X-ray picture showing the coronary circulation.

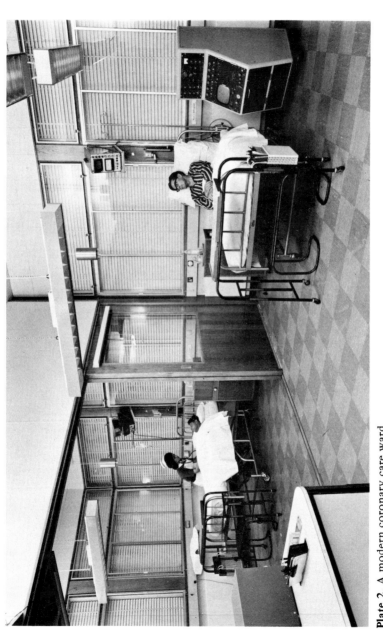

Plate 2. A modern coronary care ward.

Treatment of the coronary attack

Treatment at home

Although it has conclusively been shown that once a patient is in hospital after a heart attack he will be safer in a coronary care unit than he would be in an ordinary ward or at home, there is still some controversy as to whether all patients should be moved to hospital, as some can be successfully treated at home.

The serious complications of a coronary attack usually occur within a few hours of the onset of symptoms. In many cases the patient is not seen by a doctor within this time. The pain may come on at night, thought to be indigestion, and the doctor not called until the next morning, some hours after the attack has taken place. It could well be that the pain will have passed off by the morning so that medical help is not sought. In other cases the patient may be far from a hospital with a special coronary unit, or there may be a breakdown in the ambulance service and no means available for the transfer to hospital.

Although in uncomplicated cases where there has been no irregularity of rhythm or persisting pain after four hours the incidence of further complications is less likely, and the patient may remain at home, it must be appreciated, however, that nursing a coronary patient at home throws a considerable load both on the family and the general practitioner.

The patient should be kept in bed for the first day or two and then either remain in bed or sit in a chair at the side of the bed, whichever is the most comfortable, for the next two weeks. He should be disturbed as little as possible and visitors forbidden during this period. He should not attempt to continue his work at home and should be relieved of all business and domestic worries.

Food should be taken in bed and should be light and small in quantity with no added salt. In no circumstances should large and heavy meals be given. Fluids should be given in small amounts depending on the instructions of the doctor.

Coronary heart disease: the facts

The patient can use the lavatory if it is near the bedroom, but he should always, however, be accompanied and in no circumstances should the door be locked. If the lavatory is on a different floor or some way away from the bedroom a commode may be hired, together with a urinal.

A gradual return to activity may be undertaken over the period of two weeks, at the end of which the patient can walk around the house and then progress to short walks outside under his doctor's instructions.

It will be apparent that treating a coronary patient at home can only have a restricted application. To be successful it needs great dedication on the part of the practitioner with the use of the hospital services including electrocardiographic and blood tests. The home circumstances must be suitable for such care with a responsible person always in the house. In practice, this combination is rare, especially in urban districts. The transfer of a patient to a coronary unit relieves the family and, indeed, the patient of a great deal of worry and mental stress, especially now that people have a greater understanding of the wonderful care that is taken of the patient in a good coronary care unit.

The occurrence of further pain or the onset of irregularity of the heart's action can cause problems at home, especially if it occurs at night. Neither the patient's spouse, or whoever is looking after him, nor the patient himself will want to bother the doctor unnecessarily and thus the patient may sustain discomfort and, indeed, severe pain which would have been immediately treated in hospital. In other situations the doctor cannot be found or is so busy that he is unable to attend for some time, during which the patient may be in some severe pain or could even become unconscious.

It has been argued that the mental and physical trauma of taking a patient to hospital in an ambulance can set up complications. In reality, it is a matter of balance and judgement best left to the doctor in charge of the patient.

Treatment of the coronary attack

The coronary care unit

In the early 1960s it became increasingly recognized that patients who had suffered a coronary attack frequently developed, in the first few days of their illness, an irregularity of the heart beat, which, if treated at once, improved the patient's chance of living. From this developed the concept of the coronary care unit where the patient can be kept under constant observation by skilled nursing and medical staff and any irregularity of the heart rhythm (arrhythmia) treated by the appropriate medicine or other therapies. Most coronary care units consist of a few beds set aside in a special area or room in the hospital and are so arranged that every patient is under the constant view of the nursing staff in charge of the unit. The necessary apparatus in case of all emergencies is kept in this area (see Plate 2).

Although in some patients the site of so much electronic and other apparatus may be a little frightening, experience has shown that the constant presence of nursing and medical staff is most reassuring. It must also be emphasized that the majority of patients who have had a heart attack and are admitted to the coronary care unit need no special treatment other than rest in bed and control of any pain that they may have.

Electrocardiographic monitoring

Advances in electronics have been applied to medicine so that it is now possible to detect the minute electric currents produced in the heart, amplify them, and record them either on paper or an oscilloscope similar to a television screen. This enables the nurse or doctor to keep a continuous watch on the patient's heart beat, either at the side of the bed or relayed to a screen at the desk at which the nurse sits. Some of the more sophisticated pieces of apparatus have alarms which indicate a sudden alteration in the heart's action. On admission to the coronary unit the patient is connected to the recording apparatus (electrocardiograph) by means of wires attached to the surface of the chest by adhesive tape and wears these during his total stay in the coronary unit. Extra leads may be placed on his hands and legs when a permanent paper recording is made at regular intervals. There is, of course, no pain or discomfort associated with recording the electrocardiogram. In many cases the stay in the coronary unit of a day or two will not involve more than this, with the addition of taking of blood samples and the routine taking of blood pressure, temperature and pulse.

In some patients, as a result of the coronary attack, the heart beat may become irregular and be noticed by the patient as a 'fluttering' in the chest. Doctors can recognize many variations of these irregularities but there are basically four changes that may happen. First, the heart may occasionally miss a beat, which is recognized as a pause in the pulse at the wrist and is known as an extrasystole. Secondly, the heart rate may become excessively fast, the rapid impulse arising in one or other part of its structure and known as atrial or ventricular tachycardia. Thirdly, the heart rate may become excessively slow, known as bradycardia (the condition of 'heart block' where the electrical impulse through the heart is blocked by disease is usually associated with a slow heart rate). Fourthly, the heart's action may become totally irregular, the irregularity arising in one or the other parts of the heart and is known as atrial or ventricular fibrillation. Many of these irregularities can now be treated by suitable medicines or other means.

Nursing care

Treatment is first directed to making the patient comfortable and relieving him of any pain by morphine or similar medicines. In some cases oxygen may be given by means of a mask. This does not necessarily mean that the patient is seriously ill, but extra oxygen in the blood helps the heart to work better.

Treatment of the coronary attack

The nurse in charge of the patients in the coronary care unit has been specially trained in looking after heart patients. She takes the pulse, notes the character and rate of the breathing, and takes the temperature and blood pressure at regular intervals to detect any change in the patient's condition. The amount of fluid taken in by the patient, and that passed in the form of urine, is recorded. This is of great importance in estimating the function of the heart and kidneys.

For the first few days in the coronary unit the patient is allowed to do little for himself and he is washed and generally made comfortable by the nursing staff. He may use a commode at the side of the bed but not go to the lavatory. He is encouraged to exercise his feet and legs gently, to assist the circulation.

The diet during the first few days is light and probably without added salt. Sleep may be difficult because of worry and the strange surroundings of the hospital. A sleeping pill or tranquillizer is often given to allay fear and promote sleep. At all times it is the aim of the medical and nursing staff to keep the patient comfortable and free from pain. They are trained to listen to the patient's problems and give help and advice wherever possible.

If any irregularity of the heart is detected a small needle is placed in the vein and connected by a plastic tube to a bottle containing a weak glucose solution, which is allowed slowly to drain into the arm vein (commonly known as an 'intravenous drip'). The medicines necessary to control any irregularity can be added to the 'drip' fluid, and rapidly administered to the blood circulation. The 'wearing' of an intravenous drip is painless but may be uncomfortable from the point of view of restricting movement in bed. The most common medicine used in the drip is called 'lignocaine' but many others are available for the control of the various types of the heart's irregularity.

Coronary heart disease: the facts

Blood tests

Several changes in the composition of the blood take place as a result of injury to the heart after occlusion of one of the coronary arteries. Some of these changes are most valuable in determining whether there has, in fact, been a true coronary thrombosis.

When part of the heart is injured after thrombosis of a coronary artery the muscle affected liberates, over the course of a few days, chemical substances known as enzymes. These escape into the blood stream where they can be detected and measured. Several blood samples are taken over the period of a few days and analysed for such enzymes, which not only determine whether the patient has had a heart attack or not, but give some indication of the size of the heart injury. There are a number of enzymes which can be measured but two common ones are: creatine phosphokinase (CPK) and glutamic oxaloacetic transaminase (SGOT).

CPK is the first to rise and can be detected at the end of six hours after the attack, reaches its maximum at the end of twenty-seven hours, and then rapidly returns to normal. Some coronary units measure the iso-enzyme of CPK, which is a component of the enzyme more specific to the heart.

The level of SGOT rises less rapidly than CPK and reaches its height over the course of three to four days.

Not only the enzymes in the blood may change but also the levels of minerals, including sodium and potassium, and it is of some importance that if these should deviate from their normal levels they should be returned to the correct level by giving the appropriate medicines.

During the first few days it is common for the patient's temperature to rise for a day or more as the white blood cells increase in number to absorb and repair the injured muscle.

Complications—irregularities in the heart's rhythm

The patient's course can be divided as a general rule into the acute phase, which lasts from three to five days, and a sub-acute phase which continues while the patient remains in hospital from ten days to three weeks.

During the early hours of the attack it is not possible to say how the patient will progress. In some cases the patient remains remarkably well and suffers little discomfort or untoward symptoms and goes on to make an uninterrupted recovery.

In other cases, complications may begin to appear early in the illness. These include irregularities of rhythm of the heart (see Chapter 11), further chest pain, and failure of the heart to pump an adequate amount of blood round the circulation. It is in these cases that the organization of the coronary care unit is so valuable in enabling the right corrective treatment to be given without delay.

Irregularities in the heart's rhythm can in many cases be corrected by the use of medicines. In other cases the irregu-larity may have to be corrected either by passing an electric current through the chest (defibrillation) or by electrically stimulating the heart by means of a special soft wire inserted through a vein (pacemaking).

The cardiac defibrillator. Cardiac defibrillation has been one of the major advances in the care of heart patients and has been responsible for the saving of many thousands of lives. Patients who otherwise would have certainly died are returned to normal daily activity.

In principle the technique consists of passing a short sharp electric shock through the heart, which may be beating so irregularly that it is unable to pump enough blood round the body to maintain life. The shock often galvanizes the heart into action and corrects a serious irregularity into a normal heart beat. In the case of cardiac surgery the electric current is passed directly through the heart but a similar result can be obtained when the chest is not opened as in surgery, by placing two metal plates or electrodes on the surface of the chest. Where the patient is conscious a short anaesthetic is usually given, but should he be unconscious, this, of course, is unnecessary. The amount of electrical energy passed through the chest can be varied by dials on the apparatus from 20 to 400 watt-seconds.

The apparatus (cardiac defibrillator) for this life-saving procedure is kept in every coronary care unit.

Pacemaking in the coronary care unit. The 'pacemaker' has a special application in the coronary care unit as a temporary measure to assist the patient over an acute phase of his illness.

In some cases the 'electrical circuits' which ramify through the heart become temporarily damaged by the coronary thrombosis and do not transmit the minute electric current which is generated in the natural pacemaker of the heart. This produces the condition of 'heart block' and may cause it to beat very slowly. The treatment is artificially to 'pace' the heart by an external electric current via a fine wire which is passed into a vein of the arm or chest under a local anaesthetic and positioned into the correct part of the heart by means of an X-ray screening machine. The other end of the wire is connected to an instrument which generates a small electric current to stimulate the heart at regular intervals. In most patients in an acute coronary attack the pacing procedure can be discontinued in a few days when the heart takes over its natural function. 'Pacing' is quite painless. Pacemakers are discussed in more detail in Chapter 12.

Surgery and the acute coronary attack

Normally surgery is not indicated in the acute attack and can do little good. In the very rare case damage to the heart involving the wall between the two main chambers or ventricles of the heart may cause it to rupture and give a communication between them. In some of these patients the surgeon is able successfully to repair the hole in the heart's structure.

Treatment of the coronary attack

Drug treatment

Diuretics (water pills)

The diuretic medicines depend on their action by increasing the amount of sodium eliminated via the kidneys. This in turn encourages the removal of water from the tissues of the body and an increase in urine flow. The reduction of fluid within the circulation relieves the load on the heart and lungs and improves the breathlessness and swelling of the ankles and legs associated with cardiac disease.

Some of the diuretics not only eliminate sodium but also potassium; this is undesirable and potassium supplements (e.g. Slow K) have to be given in the form of tablets to counteract this effect.

Many types of diuretic tablets are now available varying in potency and length of time of action. The short-acting diuretics include, Saluric, Esidrex, Navidrex, Hydrenox, Frusemide, Burinex, Lasix, Moduretic, the medium-acting Aprinox, Berkoside, Brinaldix, Baycoron, Enduron, Metenix, Aquamox; and the long-acting Hygroton, Aldactone. Many of these diuretics have to be supplemented by potassium tablets but in some preparations the potassium is included in the diuretic tablet itself (e.g. Navidrex K).

Anticoagulant medicines

Since 1950 research has been directed towards finding medicines which would prevent the blood from clotting. The process of thrombosis (clotting) is extremely complex, involving many chemical and physical reactions which may be modified by drugs called 'anticoagulants'. Although these looked promising in the test tube, the early hopes that they would prevent coronary thrombosis in man were not maintained, although they have proved of great value in treating some of the complications of a heart attack. The anticoagulant medicines include the heparins, coumarin groups, and antiplatelet groups. Heparin inhibits clotting both in the test tube and in patients. It is ineffective by mouth and can only be given by injection; its action lasts a few hours. Although a valuable medicine in certain cases in hospital, it cannot be generally used unless under close medical supervision.

The coumarin group include Dindevan, Warfarin, Marevan, Sinthrome, and Tromexan, and these drugs depress the manufacture of vitamin K in the liver, which, in turn, depresses factors responsible for clotting. These medicines can be taken by mouth but the dose has to be carefully regulated by regular blood tests (the prothrombin time) to ensure that they are having the required effect. Normally a loading dose is given followed by a smaller maintenance dose. Too large a dose may lead to bleeding under the skin, in the kidneys, or in other organs. Their effect may be altered by the coincident use of other medicines, such as the barbiturates, and unexpected bleeding may occur if these are stopped.

Although at one time it was thought that taking coumarin tablets would prevent a coronary attack, there is some controversy as to their true value and many doctors do not use them for this purpose. They are, however, useful in preventing clots forming in the structures of the heart itself or in the veins of the legs rather than in the coronary arteries themselves.

At the present time anticoagulants play a useful part in preventing some of the complications of coronary heart disease but have only a weak, if any, effect on the prevention of further coronary attacks. They are prescribed for certain cases of irregularity in the heart's rhythm (atrial fibrillation) when a clot may form within the chamber of the heart, when there is clot formation in the veins of the legs or elsewhere, and after the insertion of artificial heart valves to prevent deposition of blood clots on their surface.

One of the many mechanisms of blood clotting is associated with the adherence of minute particles in the blood known as platelets (see Chapter 2). There is a group of

Treatment of the coronary attack

medicines which may, in certain circumstances, inhibit the platelets from sticking together. These include dipyridamole (Persantin), aspirin, and sulphinpyrazone (Anturan). At the present time the use of these medicines in the treatment of patients is being investigated and their exact value is not yet determined, although in certain patients they may be of benefit.

9

Recovery and rehabilitation

Few illnesses have such a psychological impact on the patient as a coronary heart attack. All those around him, including doctors, nurses, and especially his family, can help to contribute to a lasting and complete recovery both physical and mental. It should be emphasized that if the patient survives the first few hours of a heart attack he will in the majority of cases make a complete and satisfactory recovery and return to work.

When one of the arteries of the heart becomes blocked a small area of the muscle is injured and becomes inflamed and sore in a very similar way to injuries in other parts of the body. For example, if you injure your hand it hurts a great deal at first and then becomes bruised and sore. The injured part has to heal by forming a scar, a process which may take up to about six weeks. Similarly, in the injured area of the heart muscle the injured and bruised part is slowly reabsorbed and replaced by a scar. In most cases there is a firm and satisfactory repair and the reserves of the heart are such that it will perform perfectly normally. During the healing phase, however, it is desirable to keep the heart at rest as much as possible and not to throw any undue strain on it. Patients are usually kept in bed for the first week or so or, alternatively, allowed to sit quietly in a chair and to become more active towards the end of three to four weeks. From then onwards recovery is the same as in other illnesses and when the scar is firmly healed, return to work is indicated, usually a few weeks after leaving hospital.

Feelings of fear and loss of confidence are often prominent during rehabilitation from a heart attack and may continue for several months, even though the heart has recovered satisfactory. The spouse and relatives can be of immense help to the patient, especially when he returns home from hospital. Normally the patient leaves hospital two to four weeks after his heart attack, when substantial healing of the injured heart has taken place. The transition from hospital to home is often difficult, in that the patient feels the lack of protection that the hospital gives.

For the first two weeks after arriving home he should confine his activities to the house and garden. It is in order for him to walk about the house and to walk up stairs slowly but not at this stage to involve himself in heavy lifting or strenuous activity. Under no circumstances should he 'try himself out' as far as exercise is concerned, as the injury to the heart is still healing and should not be thrown under any extra strain. It has been known for patients to go to the seaside or the country, discover that they can walk quite satisfactorily for one mile on the first day, rapidly increase this distance over the course of the next few days, and have to return to hospital as a result of this too-early activity.

There is still considerable controversy among the medical profession as to the right diet, especially in relation to fats. However, all are probably agreed that it is of considerable importance that one should not over-eat on recovery from a heart attack. Large amounts of food in the stomach cause an increased flow of blood to that organ with a resultant increase in the work of the heart. Under no circumstances should the patient be encouraged to eat large amounts to 'feed him up'. Some doctors allow their patients to eat whatever they fancy providing that it is a small amount and not sufficient for them to put on weight. Other doctors believe that it is desirable to minimize the intake of animal fats, substitute polyunsaturated fats in the form of margarine and other vegetable oils for butter and lard, and increase the amount of foodstuffs containing fibre such as fresh fruit and vegetables. In all this, however, you must be guided by your own doctor. Small amounts of alcohol are not contraindicated and, in fact, if the patient is used to taking alcohol it may help him to convalesce. Excessive amounts of alcohol, however, may lead to further heart trouble, and, in some susceptible patients, may cause irregularity of its rhythm. Every effort should be made to give up smoking.

The patient's spouse and other members of the family will naturally be concerned about how to look after the patient when he returns home. It is important that he should not be fussed, and family and other worries should not be thrust upon him at an early stage. Providing that the rules outlined above are carried out, there is no reason to feel that anything further need to be done beyond maintaining a calm and peaceful atmosphere. It must be appreciated that healing from a heart attack, both physically and mentally, needs time. In many cases the patient will not be feeling himself for several weeks and, indeed, it may be up to six months before he is completely rehabilitated.

It is probably wise that sexual intercourse should not be resumed until four weeks after the heart attack and, when it is, physical exertion during the act kept to the minimum. For this purpose the side-to-side position is to be recommended and, if it is found that intercourse brings on chest pain or irregularities of the heart action associated with palpitations, it is better to not have recourse to it for a further two or three weeks. Experience has shown, however, that in the majority of patients sexual intercourse is able to be continued as before the attack.

At the end of four weeks after the attack the patient is ready to increase his activity by taking walks outside the confines of his house and garden. In the first place these should be taken slowly and for half a mile or so, increasing over the next two weeks up to three miles, providing he is free from symptoms. It is wise not to go out in very cold weather. During this time he can take rides in the car, visit a restaurant or theatre, and generally get back to a more normal way of life. He may feel tired and should not hesitate to take extra rest including an hour on his bed after lunch.

Six weeks, after the initial attack, all being well, the patient is ready to return to work. Alternatively, it might be possible to have two weeks' holiday to complete the convalescence. This time should preferably be spent quietly where it is warm.

Ideally, for the first few weeks after his return to work the patient should work half time. Many firms are agreeable to this to enable the patient to rehabilitate himself more easily. At the end of a further four weeks you should be in a position to resume normal activities.

In many cases sporting activities can be resumed at the end of two or three months after the attack. Swimming, providing the water is not too cold, or a round of golf may be beneficial. More competitive sports, such as tennis, should be treated with more caution and squash should be avoided. In recent years jogging has become fashionable as a means of preventing heart attacks but many doctors would not advise it after their patient has had a heart attack. The best form of exercise in these circumstances is probably walking or playing golf.

Some physicians recommend graded exercises under control in a gymnasium and these have proved valuable in regaining the patient's confidence and toning up muscles that have become flabby as a result of enforced idleness. There is no contra-indication to graded exercises providing they are carried out under adequate supervision, and many patients have found these helpful. Experience has shown, however, that they are not essential and that the commonsense measures of slowly increasing normal activity are adequate in most cases.

It should be reiterated that the heart cannot be strengthened by excessive exercise and, indeed, trying to do this by abnormally increasing your normal exericse may do considerable harm, especially in the first few weeks after a heart attack. The temptation to 'try yourself out' must always be rigorously resisted until healing has taken place, usually at the end of six weeks.

Minor signs and symptoms during the healing phase of a heart attack

It is inevitable that after a heart attack many patients are most apprehensive over any pains or sensations they may have in the chest following their first heart attack. During the healing phase there may be sensations associated with the healing in the heart. These include a vague aching pain or even sharp pains in the chest and there may be slight irregularities in the heart rhythm giving the sensation of missed beats. The heart may beat a little faster than expected on exercise but return to normal on rest and there may be some increased breathlessness. Tiredness, slight dizziness, and depression are not uncommon, but most of the symptoms will disappear with time.

Urgent medical help need only be called if there is severe chest pain lasting for more than half an hour, severe palpitations, or dizziness, especially if associated with short periods of unconsciousness.

After a heart attack the majority of patients are able eventually to return to work and to resume normal activities. Indeed, some patients have said that they have never felt better since their heart attack and it has been an excuse to relieve themselves of some of the heavy pressures of work and given them a new outlook on life with a better realization of how they should live.

The outlook following a coronary heart attack

The outlook following a coronary heart attack is very variable, and although an average estimate can be made for a large number of patients it is difficult to predict in the individual patient. Many patients have lived many years

Recovery and rehabilitation

following a severe heart attack, while others have not been so fortunate even after a mild illness.

Several research studies have been made by following the course of patients who have had heart attacks; all follow much the same pattern. Taking an overall picture and including all groups of patients, about 70 per cent are alive three years after the attack and 60 per cent at the end of six years. However the expectation of life depends greatly on factors connected with the illness. Age plays an important part and the outlook is significantly reduced in patients over 70 at the time of the attack. Congestion of the lungs and a large heart as shown on the X-ray are unfavourable factors, as is the presence of high blood pressure and diabetes. The amount of damage to the heart muscle as shown on the electrocardiogram also has a bearing on the long-term outlook. The continuation of cigarette smoking will shorten the patient's life in many cases.

With the advance of new methods of diagnosis such as the coronary angiogram it is probable that a more accurate prognosis and future of the patient's course may be given to him. Although it is prudent for anyone who has had a coronary heart attack to put his affairs in order, in many cases he will lead a long and trouble-free life and should view the future with optimism.

10

Common questions and answers about coronary heart attacks

Is a heart attack serious?

A heart attack is always serious, especially in the first few days after the attack. Because of this, special coronary care units have been set up throughout the country to ensure that there is constant medical and nursing care during this period. It is necessarily a period of some anxiety but, as each day passes, in most cases the outlook becomes progressively better. During the early stages after the heart attack you should not be unduly worried by having to deal with business or family affairs and visitors should be restricted to near relatives and then only for a short while.

How long will I have to remain in hospital or, if at home, remain in bed?

You will usually remain in hospital for between two or three weeks, although this varies according to the severity of the attack and how well you respond to treatment. Those patients who are treated at home should have two to three weeks in bed. Some doctors allow their patients to sit quietly in a chair after the first few days if this is more comfortable for the patient.

Shall I be able to return to work after my attack?

In the majority of cases you will able to resume your work, especially if it does not involve heavy physical work or driving a heavy goods or public vehicle. Coronary thrombosis is a common condition; many eminent people in public life have had heart attacks and have returned to full-time activity for a number of years.

How long will it be before I can resume work after the heart attack?

This depends to a large extent on how the injury to the heart heals but as a rough guide most people should be able to return to work at the end of six weeks. If at all possible it is helpful to return half time for the first month and very often arrangements can be made with the employers for this to be done. If the patient is reaching the age of retirement the retirement date may be brought forward, depending on the feelings both of the patient and the employer.

Shall I be able to be involved in sporting activities?

Many patients are able to resume playing golf, swimming, walking, and non-competitive tennis. Competitive sports involving considerable exercise, such as squash, should be avoided.

When can I drive again?

At the end of two months, providing driving does not produce angina pain or episodes of feeling faint due to an irregularity in the heart's rhythm.

Do I have to have a special diet?

There is still considerable controversy as to whether altering your diet after a heart attack in middle or late age has any effect on the arteries. Large meals should be avoided but there is no harm in having small amounts of whatever food gives the most pleasure. It is important that you should not put on weight and that if you are already obese a reducing diet should be instituted. Some doctors believe that animal fats should be avoided and there is certainly no harm in this and it may do good. Perhaps the rule should be 'moderation in all things'.

Is smoking harmful?

All doctors agree that heavy smokers are more liable to have heart attacks and that if you continue to smoke after a heart attack you are more likely to have another. Tobacco smoke contains a high proportion of carbon monoxide, which combines with the blood and prevents the proper oxygenation of the tissues; this can damage the cells lining the arteries and produce further heart attacks. The nicotine may contribute to the irregularity in the heart's action and in extreme cases lead to very serious illness or death.

Can I have a drink?

There is no good evidence to show that alcohol in moderation has an effect on the incidence of heart attacks. Excessive drinking, however, should be avoided. A glass of sherry or whisky before dinner, and a glass of wine with the meal is often good for your morale. There are a few patients, however, whose hearts are sensitive to alcohol and this may bring on irregularities of the heart action recognized as palpitations. If these are noted, then alcohol should be avoided.

Can I climb stairs?

In the majority of cases there is no reason why, after the end of four weeks, you should not climb stairs slowly. The work involved in doing this is relatively small and will do no harm.

Coronary heart attack—common questions

You should not, however, attempt to try yourself out by running up stairs but take them slowly. If you find this unduly tiring, have a rest half way up. Only in a very few cases is it necessary to move a bed into a downstairs room permanently.

When can I have sexual intercourse?

Providing you have made an uninterrupted recovery, sexual intercourse may be resumed at the end of six weeks, as long as it is not associated with too much exertion, and does not provoke chest pain. Sexual activity in association with a large meal, or excessive drinking or smoking should be avoided, at least for a few months after the heart attack.

May I lift heavy weights?

Heavy strenuous exercise, such as lifting heavy weights, digging, pushing the car, or shovelling snow should be avoided for several months after the heart attack.

How much exercise should I take?

The best form of exercise after a heart attack is probably walking. Short, gentle walks may usually be started four to five weeks after the attack. In no circumstances, however, should you try yourself out to see how much exercise you are able to take without incurring symptoms. In many cases this will lead to further damage to the heart before the injury has properly healed. The amount of exercise should be slowly increased over a period of a few months starting with a half-a-mile walk on the flat. It is not possible to strengthen the heart by exercise before the injury has healed, although you can slowly tone-up the muscles of the legs and the rest of the body by gentle exercises.

Coronary heart disease: the facts

Some doctors advocate that the patient should go to a gymnasium for rehabilitation. Providing that is carried out under full medical supervision there is no harm in this and it may improve your morale and general well-being.

When can I travel after a heart attack?

Quite often the patient has a heart attack away from home or away on holiday and in these circumstances wishes to go home as soon as possible. If there are no complications it is usually possible for him to return home at the end of approximately three weeks, preferably in a car, and to limit the length of the journey in any one day to 200 miles.

Can I fly?

If you have a heart attack far from home or in a foreign country, you may fly home at the end of three weeks providing the airline agrees and arrangements are made to put you on the plane in a wheelchair, to have oxygen available in the aircraft, and to meet you at the other end by a car. Flying to go on holiday can usually be safely undertaken at the end of eight weeks but you should be accompanied by spouse or friend who can make the arrangements at the airport and not allow you to carry heavy luggage.

It must be remembered, when arranging a holiday, that the medical facilities will not be the same as those available at home; if any further trouble should happen you may regret having gone so far. Convalescence is probably better spent not too far from home or where adequate medical care is available.

What should I do if I have further chest pain?

Vague aches and pains are common for a few months after a heart attack and may safely be ignored. Some patients are left with anginal pain which usually lasts for a minute or two and then passes off and is relieved by a trinitrin tablet placed under the tongue. If the pain is not relieved by the trinitrin and persists for more than twenty minutes seek medical help.

Is it usual to experience palpitations and what can be done if they occur?

The occasional 'missed beat' or palpitation is not uncommon after a heart attack and can be ignored. Prolonged palpitations, or a very slow heart-rate under 45 beats a minute, call for treatment by appropriate therapeutic methods and medical help should be sought.

Why am I short of breath?

Some shortness of breath is common in the early stages of a heart attack because of excess fluid in the lungs. This is usually treated by diuretics (water pills) and rapidly improves. During the period of rehabilitation over six months any residual breathlessness usually improves. Your doctor should be consulted if there are episodes of severe breathlessness at night at these may call for more vigorous treatment by diuretics.

Why do I feel tired or depressed?

The period following a heart attack is a stressful time, both physical and mental, in a person's life and a time of readjustment to new circumstances and self-evaluation. Feelings of tiredness or depression are common, but experience has shown that matters improve week by week for the first few months when the necessary mental adjustments have been made. Not infrequently a patient finds in retrospect that a heart attack has enabled him to realize true values with a consequent greater enjoyment of life.

Coronary heart disease: the facts

Will I always have to take tablets?

In most patients a firm scar forms in the heart wall after a heart attack and no further treatment is necessary. Where angina persists it may be necessary to take tablets regularly. Recently, research has shown that beta-blocking drugs, aspirin, and sulphinpyrazone may possibly have some place in the prevention of a further heart attack. This work is in an early stage and the nuisance of taking these drugs and their side-effects may outweigh the theoretical advantages.

Is heart disease hereditary?

There is evidence that heart disease tends to occur in families, as does high blood pressure. If there is a family history then there is a greater likelihood of relatives developing heart disease. This, however, is only an increased likelihood and does not mean for certain that anyone will have a heart attack. It is prudent, however, if you have a bad family history, not to add the other risk factors, such as smoking and obesity.

What can I do to prevent a further heart attack?

At the present time a great deal of research is being carried out in the field of prevention. All authorities are agreed that smoking increases the likelihood of a further attack, and that loss of weight may be beneficial, but there is still controversy about diet. A moderate amount of exercise can do no harm and may be beneficial. Adequate sleep and the avoidance of undue stress may also help.

More recently new treatments have been introduced for which claims have been made that they reduce the likelihood of a further attack. These include small doses of aspirin and sulphinpyrasone (Anturan). Their efficacy has yet to be established.

11

Irregularities in the rhythm of the heart

In health, at rest, the heart beats regularly at approximately 60–90 beats a minute, as can be felt in the pulse at the wrists. During exercise or excitement the rate may increase up to 150 beats a minute.

The electrical impulse for the activation of the heart beat is normally generated in a small collection of cells known as the sino-atrial node. This structure covers an area in the atrium of the heart of only a few square millimetres and is surrounded by nerve endings of the 'autonomic' nervous system. This system is responsible for controlling bodily activities that are carried out unconsciously and regulates the rate at which the sino-atrial node discharges. For example, when you are excited or nervous the brain passes messages to the sino-atrial node which causes it to operate at a faster rate so that the heart itself beats faster. The action of the sino-atrial node can also be affected by medicinal drugs.

The electrical impulse generated by the sino-atrial node passes down specialized fibres to all parts of the heart causing it to contract rhythmically. The main bundle of fibres is known as the atrioventricular bundle or 'bundle of His', the name of the man who first described it.

In coronary arterial disease any of these electrical structures may be affected and either lead to a disturbance in heart-rate or inco-ordination of the normal contraction of the heart. Irregularity of the heart beat is very common in the acute stage following a heart attack.

Sick sinus syndrome

With partial failure of the sino-atrial node as an electrical generator there may be intermittent periods when the heart goes very slowly followed by other periods when it beats rapidly (the sick sinus syndrome). Although the symptoms associated with the sick sinus syndrome are often unpleasant and can be corrected, if severe, by the insertion of an artificial pacemaker, recent researches have shown that patients with this illness have exactly the same outlook as far as mortality is concerned as the rest of the population.

Tachycardia

With a complete failure of the sino-atrial node another focus of electrical generation in the atrium of the heart may take over, causing the heart to beat at a very fast rate (tachycardia). If this focus is situated in the atrium the resultant fast heart-rate is known as a 'supraventricular tachycardia'. The atrium may be stimulated up to 350 times a minute in a regular fashion (atrial tachycardia or atrial flutter). As the rate of stimulation increases, the contractions become chaotic and are then known as atrial fibrillation. This is perhaps analogous to the escapement mechanism of a clock which can lose control and cause the mechanism to whirr away at a fast rate.

These irregularities of the heart's rhythm can usually be successfully controlled by medicines or, in selected cases, by the passage of an electric shock through the patient's chest, under an anaesthetic.

Missed beats (extrasystoles)

Extrasystoles, or the sensation of the heart missing a beat, are not uncommon in otherwise healthy people but probably more common in patients with coronary heart disease. Either at regular or irregular intervals the patient notices a vague sensation in his chest and perhaps a thumping over the heart

64

itself. Some describe the sensation 'as though the heart was turning over', others 'as though the heart stops'. If the extrasystoles are frequent, they give the sensation of palpitations. In many cases extrasystoles are harmless and the exact cause of their origin is unknown. Often they only come on at night and may wake the patient from sleep.

Extrasystoles may be associated with drinking alcohol and appear several hours after drinking, possibly because of the breakdown products of the alcohol in the body. In other patients tea and coffee in excess or smoking may be the culprits in the production of extrasystoles. When they are relatively infrequent they can be ignored. If, however, they become frequent during the whole of the 24 hours medical advice should be sought, as they can often be controlled by taking an appropriate medicine.

Heart block

The electrical impulses generated in the sino-atrial node pass in an ordered fashion though the special conducting circuits to all parts of the heart. In coronary arterial disease part of this conducting system may be injured and thus the electric currents are blocked from reaching all parts of the heart. This condition is known as 'heart block'.

Heart block may be temporary after a coronary attack, where there is bruising and swelling of the muscle of the heart which may temporarily interfere with the normal conduction through the specialized circuits. With healing the situation reverses. In other cases it becomes permanent because the disease process is more advanced. Heart block can be complete, when all the connections are involved, or partial when either the connections to the right side of the heart (right bundle branch block) or to the left side (left bundle branch block) are affected.

Complete heart block usually leads to a very slow heart-rate—around 35–45 beats a minute—and often the heart may stop beating for a few seconds. Some patients with heart block have few symptoms, while others may have attacks of dizziness or unconsciousness (Stokes–Adams attacks, named after the physicians who described them first in the 1830s). The attacks of unconsciousness may be associated with pallor of the skin, followed by flushing when the patient comes round. These attacks may be helped to some extent by medicines (isoprenaline or Saventrine) but recent advances in the science of electrically pacing the heart have revolutionized the treatment of complete heart block and nowadays patients with this condition can lead active lives free from all symptoms and discomfort.

Right and left bundle branch blocks diagnosed by the electrocardiogram are not usually associated with specific symptoms and need no special treatment. Right bundle branch block is found in otherwise normal people and in these cases can be ignored. Left bundle branch block is more often associated with coronary artery disease, which in itself may need treatment.

Irregularities of ventricular rhythm

In some patients irregularities of the rhythm of the heart may originate in the muscles of the ventricular wall of the heart. The exact mechanism of their production is unknown but they are associated with a rapid beating of the heart either in a regular (ventricular tachycardia) or grossly irregular form (ventricular fibrillation). Both are not uncommon after an acute coronary attack.

In ventricular tachycardia the ventricles suddenly start beating very rapidly up to a rate of 300 beats a minute, possibly initiated by an abnormal electrical impulse in the damaged ventricle itself. When the heart beats very quickly it becomes inefficient as a pump, as there is not time between beats for it to fill. It is therefore unable to maintain an adequate circulation. Tachycardia may be accompanied by dizziness or attacks of unconsciousness resulting from the compromised circulation. In some cases ventricular tachycardia may be treated effectively with medicines alone. Such treatment often has to be carried out on a 'trial and error' basis, as the doctor has several medicines at his disposal to which individual patients respond differently. In many cases ventricular tachycardia may present as an emergency. Under these curcumstances an electric shock is given by the cardiac defibrillator.

Until relatively recently ventricular fibrillation, a condition in which the ventricles of the heart beat very rapidly in a totally uncoordinated way, was almost invariably fatal. Modern advances in medical research have changed all this and many patients who otherwise would certainly have died have been restored to continue a normal life. Ventricular fibrillation invariably leads to a loss of consciousness and, if left without treatment, to death. A very few patients can be restored to a regular rhythm by a sharp blow on the front of the chest but most need electrical defibrillation by direct current countershock, which forms the basis for cardiac resuscitation described in a separate chapter.

12

Pacemakers

Coronary artery disease is occasionally associated with an interference with the blood supply to the sino-atrial node electrical pacemaker in the heart and the special cells that conduct the tiny electric current through its structures which cause it to contract at the right rate and in the right sequence. Although coronary arterial disease is one of the main causes of the electrical disturbance, there may be disruption by other diseases or by congenital abnormalities.

The symptoms produced by a failing sinus node (the heart's natural pacemaker) may include a sudden slowing of the heart followed by episodes of rapid regular, or irregular, beating, either of which may be accompanied by dizziness, faintness, or even short periods of unconsciousness.

If the connections between the pacemaker and the rest of the heart are interrupted, the electrical impulse cannot reach the ventricles and initiate their contraction. This is known as heart block, which can be intermittent or permanent. Fortunately in many cases an 'emergency pacemaker' situated in the lower part of the conducting system takes over at a slow rate in the region of 30–45 beats a minute. However, the heart may stop beating for a few seconds and be accompanied by an attack of unconsciousness (Stokes–Adams attacks) or at least by a sensation of faintness or giddiness.

Some relief may be obtained by medicines such as isoprenaline (or Saventrin) but remarkable advances have been made in the treatment of this condition by the introduction of electrical pacing, or stimulating the heart by an artificial pacemaker.

The development of this method is an example of medical and scientific research applied to the relief of disease, and, indeed, to the saving of life. In the late 1940s experiments were carried out to see whether the heart could be stimulated by passing an intermittent electric current through the surface of the chest, and several patients with heart block were treated in this way. Unfortunately, the strength of the current necessary to stimulate the heart was such that it also caused painful contractions of the muscles of the chest wall. Some years previously, however, a German surgeon, Forsmann, had shown that he could safely pass a tube through a vein in the arm into his heart. He performed this experiment on himself by watching the passage of the tube through his body in a mirror reflecting the image on an X-ray machine. This pioneering work opened up the whole field of cardiac catheterization (passing tubes and wires into the heart), for which he received the Nobel Prize.

The next step in the development of cardiac pacing was to insert a fine wire under X-ray control through a vein in the arm or chest and place its end in contact wiht the inside of the heart. The other end was connected to a box which contained the necessary electronic apparatus to give the rhythmic currents to stimulate the heart. This was a great step forward in treating the patient who was confined to bed but there were still problems: the patient's activities were restricted, as he was connected to an external machine, and infection and inflammation occurred around the site of insertion of the wire. The original electronic boxes were large and powered by thermonic valves which drew a large current and could never be inserted into the patient's body. Through research connected with space travel, the invention of transistors and the silicon chip has led to miniaturization of the electronic stimulator, which is now the size of a small matchbox. The box is so small that it can easily be inserted under the skin and remain there without discomfort for several years.

The implantable pacemaker today consists of an electrical pulse generator connected to a fine wire in contact with the heart. The generator is an encapsulated unit made of an inert metal which totally seals the electronic components. It is made of two parts: the electronic circuit and the batteries. The electronic circuits are of varying types and used according to the patient's disease. Some give a fixed impulse, while others automatically switch in only when the patient's own heart rate falls below a certain pre-set figure.

For some time the batteries were of the mercury type which had a limited life of only a year or two and in some cases failed suddenly without warning. Recent research has developed the lithium battery which usually has a life span of seven years or more. Atomic-powered pacemakers have also been developed with an even longer life but they are more expensive and safeguards against radiation and disposal after the death of the patient have given them a limited use. With the development of the lithium cell there is little advantage in their use. Some years ago a pacemaker using an induction coil on the surface of the chest was developed but subsequent designs have now made this obsolete.

Implantation of the pacemaker

Several methods are at present in use for implanting the pacemaker into a patient's body but usually one of two main procedures are used, depending on the patient's medical history and the surgeon's preference. These are known as the endocardial and epicardial routes. In the former a wire is passed into the inside of the heart, and, in the latter, wires are sewn on to the outside of the heart.

The endocardial method is performed either under a local or general anaesthetic. A fine, soft wire is passed through a vein in the armpit or neck and its tip, on which there is a small electrode, is positioned against the wall of the right ventricle under the control of an X-ray screen where it may be seen by the operator. An incision is made in the chest wall and a small pouch is formed in the tissues overlying the wall into which the pacemaker generator is placed and connected to the wire to the heart. The incision in the chest wall is then stitched up and when healed there should be no further discomfort.

When the epicardial route is used the operation is performed under a general anaesthetic, and the surgeon makes a small incision in the abdomen just below the chest wall, sews the electrode on the surface of the heart, and then implants the pacemaker generator in the wall of the abdomen.

These operations are quite safe. Afterwards the patient stays a few days in hospital until the wound has healed.

Pacemakers and external electrical sources of interference

Modern pacemakers have been designed and shielded to be extremely resistant to interference by external sources of electrical radiation. Susceptibility varies among different makes and the manufacturer's instructions have to be followed by the doctor in charge in his advice to his patient. Potential sources of interference include close proximity to radar and amateur radio transmitters, microwave ovens, and diathermy apparatus used by surgeons. The security screening apparatus used at airports might also affect the pacemaker function in the isolated case.

However all this should not cause any worry because the patient should become aware of a change in his heart rate and move away from the source of radiation. In practice these sort of problems practically never occur.

The aftercare of the pacemaker patient

The great majority of pacemaker patients live a normal and trouble-free life as far as the pacemaker is concerned. However, the functioning of the pacemaker should be checked every 6–12 months. Advanced apparatus enables doctors precisely to test the functioning of the generator and the state of the batteries merely by connecting two electrocardiographic electrodes to the arms.

13

Surgery and coronary heart disease

The remarkable advances in the development of open heart surgery, during which the heart may be disconnected from the arteries and veins and an artificial circulation substituted, has led to major advances in treatment of heart disease by surgical means.

Coronary artery bypass grafting

Two main arteries from the aorta supply the heart: one on the left side and one on the right; the artery on the left quickly divides into two and may become blocked before its division (left main stem) or after it has separated into two.

Blocked arteries can be replaced by lengths of vein from the leg. Although it still has to be established that, apart from a few well-defined exceptions, surgery of the coronary arteries increases the length of life, there is no doubt that in many patients it relieves the symptoms of pain.

The surgical procedure is carried out by connecting the circulation to the heart–lung machine and arresting the action of the patient's heart, usually by means of a paralysing fluid. A length of vein is then taken from the leg and connected from the aorta to the coronary artery beyond the position where it is blocked. This is a very delicate operation as each end of the vein has to be securely sewn to the other blood vessels. Occasionally, veins may be taken from other areas of the body. One, two, three, or even four of these grafts may be inserted, depending on the severity of the disease.

The risks associated with the operation are remarkably small and in skilled hands the mortality may be as low as 1–2 per cent. It is, however, an operation which can be

Surgery and coronary heart disease

performed only in specialized centres and demands the highest surgical skill, both from the surgeon himself and from the nursing staff during the period of intensive care immediately after the operation. Convalescence may take up to three months.

The operation is generally confined to the 'low-risk' patients, who are less than 70 years old, have a normal size heart with a good function, and have had no recent evidence of a heart attack and no co-existing adverse medical diseases. The coronary arteries, themselves, must be suitable for grafting, and this can be shown by angiography.

The main result of the surgery is improvement of angina pectoris in about 90 per cent of the patients. In about two-thirds of patients the angina disappears completely and, in some cases, improves breathlessness too. The improvement often directly improves quality of life and working capacity, although there is no guaranteee that the symptoms will not eventually return or that the patient will not have a heart attack.

Various tests of the function of the heart itself after such surgery have not conclusively shown an improvement. Although there is a tendency for the replaced veins in the heart to become involved in the disease process themselves, something like 80 per cent have been reported to be still open one year after the operation in the most experienced centres. Further occlusions of the graft are relatively rare and average about 2 per cent annually.

A working group of physicians and surgeons established by the World Health Organization has laid down the following as indications for coronary artery surgery in suitable patients.

(1) stable or unstable angina when there is an obstruction of 50 per cent or more in the left main coronary artery, and

(2) stable angina pectoris, sufficient to impair substantially the individual's usual level of activity, which has not responded to adequate medical treatment over a period of several months. 'Adequate medical treatment' includes the correct use of the full therapeutic range of

beta-adrenergic blocking agents and other anti-anginal compounds, as well as treatment of conditions such as obesity, hypertension, anaemia, and heart failure. In addition, the patient's life-style should be adjusted so that he had adequate physical exercise and rest and avoids sudden massive exertion and psychological stress. He should stop smoking.

(3) A third indication is unstable angina pectoris where the angina is increasing in frequency, duration, or severity, including pain at rest, and pain not responding to adequate medical therapy, and excluding acute myocardial infarction.

The other indications for cardiac surgery are for the treatment of the complications of coronary thrombosis. These include the repair of the hole produced between the chambers of the heart by rupture of the muscle (ventricular septal defect), and repair of heart valves where their attachment to the muscle of the heart has been damaged.

Recent years have seen the development of the 'balloon pump', which is an elaborate apparatus consisting of an elastic inflatable sac on the end of a flexible tube that can be inserted into the main blood vessel of the heart (aorta) through the artery in the leg. Once in position, rhythmic inflation of the 'balloon' augments the action of the heart. The main value of this machine is to improve the patient's condition if surgery of the heart has to be undertaken as an emergency.

The demand for heart surgery

The incidence of angina in a typical British general practice is shown in Table 1. From this it can be extrapolated that

Table 1 Incidence of angina in typical British general practice

Patients	(no.)
Total no.	2500
With angina	20
With hypertension	25
With heart failure	30

0.8 per cent of the population have angina. Of these it is assumed that approximately 10 per cent of subjects with angina will have symptoms sufficiently severe to warrant an operation. This assumption is based more on consensus of opinion than on hard data. The proportion of patients needing surgery is higher for those with angina following a heart attack—so-called post-infarction angina (Table 2).

Table 2 Estimate of annual need for surgery in new and post-infarct angina patients

	New angina	Post-infarct angina
Total with angina	400	100
Warranting operation	40	25
Incremental from previous years	40	—
Angina not sufficient to dictate surgery, but damage to heart muscle present	20	—
Total cases requiring surgery per year	100	25

125 new male cases of angina develop each year per million population. The proportion of females developing angina is smaller—perhaps 20 per cent of the incidence in males— a figure consistent with the typical fraction of current surgical cases. The total number of new patients meriting surgery for relief of severe angina is thus approximately 150 per annum per million population.

Against this background must be considered the resources available for the operation. The cost of coronary artery investigation and surgery provided by several centres in Europe has been estimated at about £5000 per patient within a range of £2500–£7500 a patient. Most private patients cannot afford this sum unless they are adequately insured, and thus a considerable load is thrown on the National Health Service.

From the patient's point of view the relief of pain is the main benefit and in many cases this will permit the return to work of those who otherwise would have been unemployed. On the other hand, it must be appreciated that medical treatment may achieve similar results but at the same time this involves long-continued expense in the provision of medicines.

14

Diet and heart disease

Throughout the ages doctors have believed that many diseases were partly caused by diet. In the past there was good reason for this belief, as food was often deficient in essential vitamins and other substances that are needed to maintain adequate health. Thus scurvy, which was such a scourge in the Navy, was found to be due to lack of vitamin C and was totally cured when lime juice was introduced into the diet of sailors in the eighteenth century. Rickets was shown to be caused by lack of vitamin D and other diseases were associated with the lack of other vitamins. Under-nutrition resulted in poor growth and general ill-health of the poorer population in times past.

Today it is unlikely that most of us in the western world are suffering from any deficiency disease. On the contrary, the modern problem is that of over-eating, starting with children being encouraged to eat an excessive quantity of food, and later, social entertainment being arranged around the consumption of food, whether it be the business lunch, afternoon tea parties, or dinner functions. Modern man tends, on the whole, to eat more than he really needs for his body to function properly. Not only does excessive food overload the normal functions of the body but it lays down fat in our fat cells so that we become overweight and as a result have to carry an extra load. This can be compared to walking around, climbing stairs, and performing all one's normal activities holding two heavy suitcases in your hand. If your heart is in any way affected by disease it is even more important to avoid carrying this extra load, and you certainly do not need 'feeding up' during your convalescence from a heart attack.

Insurance companies' statistics have conclusively shown that being more than 20 per cent overweight shortens life expectancy. Excessive weight exacerbates arthritic hips and varicose veins, and an obese patient is at a higher risk from surgical operations. It is, therefore, prudent, even without heart disease, to keep one's weight within normal limits. Ideally one should have no excessive fat, and this you can test most easily when you are lying in the bath by picking up the folds in your abdomen. The fat is useless as far as your health is concerned and, indeed, is often harmful. Table 3 shows *average* weights for various heights and ages; *desirable* weight for each height is the average weight shown for age less than 30.

Excessive fat is only produced by eating more than your body needs. Over-eating is a matter of habit to a large extent, although many people use food as a form of tranquillizer and

Table 3 Average weight (lb) in relation to height and age

Height	Under 30 Men	Under 30 Women	30–39* Men	30–39* Women	40–49* Men	40–49* Women	50–59* Men	50–59* Women	60+* Men	60+* Women	Height
4'11"	–	115	–	121	–	128	–	131	–	133	4'11"
5 ft.	–	117	–	123	–	130	–	133	–	135	5 ft.
5'1"	–	119	–	125	–	132	–	136	–	138	5'1"
5'2"	–	121	–	127	–	135	–	139	–	142	5'2"
5'3"	134	124	138	130	141	138	142	142	139	145	5'3"
5'4"	136	127	142	134	145	141	146	145	143	148	5'4"
5'5"	141	131	146	138	149	145	150	149	146	152	5'5"
5'6"	144	134	150	142	154	149	155	152	152	154	5'6"
5'7"	148	138	154	146	158	153	159	157	156	159	5'7"
5'8"	151	142	158	150	162	157	163	162	161	164	5'8"
5'9"	156	146	163	154	167	161	168	166	166	168	5'9"
5'10"	160	150	167	158	171	164	173	171	171	175	5'10"
5'11"	165	154	172	160	176	168	178	175	176	179	5'11"
6 ft.	170	158	176	164	180	171	182	179	181	186	6 ft.
6'1"	175	–	181	–	185	–	187	–	186	–	6'1"
6'2"	179	–	186	–	190	–	192	–	191	–	6'2"
6'3"	183	–	192	–	196	–	198	–	197	–	6'3"

*Note: *Desirable* weights are roughly equivalent to average weights under 30.

5 feet = 1.524 metres; 1 kg = 2.21 lbs; 100 lbs = 45 kg

eat to give themselves some comfort. As with other habits the habit of over-eating is far from easy to break, and, indeed, society is to some extent organized to produce obesity in its members. However, those who have had a heart attack or have angina in particular should lose weight to relieve symptoms and prolong life. The way to do it is to develop the habit of eating less and of eating bulky foods which are not absorbed and so do not lay down fat. Crash courses to try and lose weight over a few weeks are usually ineffective in the long run and any weight that may be lost is rapidly regained. It is much better slowly to get into the habit of eating less food and to learn what foods you may eat which in themselves do not lead to excessive obesity.

The habit developed over the last few hundred years of eating three large meals a day is probably excessive. Dogs stay in excellent health by eating one meal a day without any snacks between. It is probably likely that man needs only one large meal a day with perhaps a small amount of food for the other two. Certainly a large lunch *and* a large dinner are entirely unnecessary for the maintenance of good health.

A good way to start losing weight is to develop the habit of not eating food of any sort, including snacks, biscuits, nuts, etc., between meals. When this habit is established arrange to have half the amount of your usual serving of food on the plate, eat slowly, and in no circumstances have a second helping. Breakfast should be restricted to one piece of toast with marmalade and an apple with coffee. Next decide whether you want to have your main meal at lunchtime or in the evening. The other meal can be made up cheese and biscuits with some fruit. In this way you can slowly wean yourself from the habit of over-eating and so considerably improve your general health.

At the same time as introducing these new habits, you should become aware of the food stuffs that make you put on excessive weight. These include sugar, chocolate, jam, honey and marmalade, all fried foods, butter, other fats, cream, margarine, dried or condensed milk, ice cream, sausages, salad cream and other bought sauces, biscuits, cakes, pastry, and puddings containing flour or sugar, bread (especially white), and pasta. Alcohol, especially beer, is very high in calories and is fattening, as are sweetened drinks including tonic water. Nuts, crisps, and cocktail snacks should be avoided.

Eat more fresh fruit, green salads and vegetables, wholemeal bread, high protein foods such as fresh meat (without fat), chicken, fish and skimmed milk, but, above all, eat smaller amounts at meal times and nothing between meals.

Another way of losing weight has been devised by the Weight Watchers organization. They have selected food stuffs which you can eat without putting on weight so that, during the weight reduction course, you can eat as much of these as you like. The organization keeps a very firm eye on what is happening to your weight and supports and encourages you when this is needed. Many patients have found that joining Weight Watchers is very helpful. However, in the long run it is a matter of developing new eating habits, with support from the family, so that you actually eat less.

Doctors are often asked by their patients to prescribe pills which will reduce their appetite and help them to lose weight. Although these pills are available they have undesirable side-effects and you certainly cannot use them over a long period of time.

We do not yet know whether changing the constituents of your diet in adult life really helps to prevent coronary heart disease. Some authorities recommend the substitution of polyunsaturated (margarine, vegetable oils) for saturated fatty acids (animal fats) but an expert panel of the Department of Health and Social Security were unanimous in remaining unconvinced by the available evidence that the incidence of coronary heart disease would be reduced as a result of a rise in the ratio of polyunsaturated to saturated fatty acids in the diet. The same panel did recommend, however, that there should be an overall reduction of all fats in the diet and that sugar should be reduced to prevent obesity.

It should be pointed out, however, that excessive worry about food can spoil one's enjoyment of life and in itself lead to nervous disorders. The best advice is to eat whatever you fancy but only in small amounts. If you are willing to alter your diet reduce the amount of fat, and avoid food that puts on weight.

For advice on minimizing other risk factors associated with heart disease, see Chapter 4.

15

Driving and coronary heart disease

Heart attacks and strokes are responsible for more than one-half of the deaths every year in the United Kingdom. These may occur without warning and often lead to sudden collapse. Many men spend an hour a day, or 4 per cent of their middle-aged life, driving a motor car, and it is not surprising that some of them collapse from heart attacks in the driver's seat. To what extent then is this disease a risk to road safety?

All forms of sudden illness combined are probably responsible for about 1 accident per 1000 reportable accidents. Collapse from coronary heart disease (non-fatal and fatal) appears to account for one-sixth to one-seventh of sudden illness accidents. Heart attacks causing collapse or sudden death in the driver's seat and the consequences have been the subject of a number of reports, and there are two series of particular interest. In one series, of 81 sudden deaths at the wheel, coronary heart disease was responsible in three-quarters of them. Accidents followed 36 of the 81 deaths (44 per cent) causing damage to property and injury to pedestrians, passengers, or other drivers. During the same period of time that the 81 fatalities were recorded, 24 persons collapsed and died of natural causes while they were passengers in cars or buses: in 20 (83 per cent) of them the cause was coronary heart disease. In another series of 52 deaths at the wheel of private cars, 20 (38 per cent) drivers were unable to stop and avoid major accidents.

The evidence in these reports is in keeping with the experience of many cardiologists—that persons who develop severe and even fatal coronary attacks while driving may have sufficient warning to slow down or stop before losing consciousness. Tragic exceptions have occasionally occurred, however, resulting in severe injury and death to other drivers and pedestrians. Coronary heart disease poses a driving risk, but a small one, considering the number of coronary patients who drive cars. It is certainly not serious enough to warrant disqualifying all of them, but some are believed to be at particular risk and should not drive.

Patients are advised not to drive:

(1) within two months after clinical recovery from a coronary thrombosis (myocardial infarction), and thereafter they should notify the Licensing Centre of their condition;

(2) when angina pectoris is easily provoked during driving, either by the mechanical act of driving, or by the annoyance caused by other drivers or by everyday city driving conditions (if you are an experienced driver with a long history of angina provoked only by unusual or avoidable effort you need not be advised against driving),

(3) if you are liable to arrhythmias (irregular heart action).

A stable and controlled arrhythmia, such as atrial fibrillation, is not a driving hazard. Paroxysmal arrhythmias (intermittent irregularities) can be, since the ventricular rate may be fast. A relatively small number of persons describe weakness, light-headedness, or visual blurring during a prolonged attack and, in middle-aged or elderly persons, anginal pain may appear. In these, driving is unwise if the attacks are frequent.

If you have an implanted pacemaker, and are under continual medical supervision, and can produce a supporting letter from a cardiologist indicating that your pacemaker is functioning normally and is likely to continue to do so for a further year, you may be allowed to drive, provided you notify the Licensing Centre.

Coronary heart disease: the facts

Heavy goods vehicles and public service vehicles

A more uniform and generally stricter procedure relating to heart disease is followed for drivers of heavy goods vehicles and public service vehicles. Coronary heart disease provides the greatest risk, and sudden collapse at the wheel in these categories of drivers may result in grave injury to other drivers, pedestrians, and property. Over a period of 20 years, eight London Transport bus drivers collapsed and became unconscious from coronary heart disease while driving and were unable to stop, serious accidents occurring in six instances. Twenty-four others became acutely ill at the wheel from coronary heart disease. While these figures emphasize the need for special health standards for public service vehicle drivers, they represent only a very small threat to public safety, for during the 20 years there were 334 000 man years of driving experience and 6300 million miles were driven.

A person is advised not to apply for or to hold a licence to drive a heavy goods or public service vehicle in the following circumstances:

(1) If he is subject to anginal pain, whether this is brought on by slight or energetic exercise or emotion, or meals, or if it awakes him from sleep. An exercise electrocardiographic test should be carried out when the identity of a chest pain is in doubt; if signs of coronary disease develop, driving should not be permitted;
(2) if he has had a coronary thrombosis (myocardial infarction) in the past, however remote, or however complete his recovery;
(3) if his electrocardiogram (ECG) shows any of the accepted stigmata of coronary heart disease, regardless of the absence of corresponding symptoms,
(4) if the electrocardiogram is abnormal, apart from the abnormalities mentioned above, particularly if it shows left bundle branch block or complete heart block. Right bundle branch block should be regarded in the same light if it occurs after a previously recorded normal ECG or is detected for the first time after the age of 40, or when associated with chest pain, diabetes, or hypertension. Other non-specific abnormalities of the electrocardiogram should be carefully appraised including a submaximal effort test;
(5) if significant enlargement of the heart is found on X-ray examination;

(6) if there is a history of or if the electrocardiogram shows an arrhythmia (irregularity in the heart's rhythm);

(7) if casual blood-pressure readings are 200/110 or over. Persons whose hypertension is effectively controlled by diuretics and beta-adrenergic blockers may be accepted but drivers undergoing treatment with more potent hypotensive drugs should normally be rejected;

(8) if he is the subject of fainting attacks or unexplained attacks of unconsciouness;

(9) if a cardiac pacemaker has been implanted.

If any part of the cardiovascular system is suspect in a heavy goods or public service vehicle driver, a yearly examination should be carried out.

16

Flying and coronary heart disease

The airline passenger travels in a somewhat different environment from that on the ground. As far as healthy individuals are concerned this has little effect but patients with heart trouble may be at a disadvantage. The modern airliner operates at altitudes between 25 000 and 40 000 feet, which is above turbulence and adverse weather and so makes for a smooth and fast passage. Because of the height, the cabin has to be pressurized to maintain an adequate concentration of oxygen. For technical reasons it is not possible to produce a pressure equal to that found at sea level. In practice some reduction of cabin pressure is acceptable and most modern airliners operate with a cabin pressure range equivalent to altitudes of 5000–7000 feet above sea-level, up to a ceiling of 8000 feet.

At 6000 feet above sea-level the reduction in atmospheric pressure may cause gas trapped in body cavities to expand and give trouble with the ears or sinuses, or cause abdominal discomfort. This, although it may be unpleasant, has no serious implications.

Patients with serious heart disease may be adversely affected by the lowered amount of oxygen in the air in the carbin. Fortunately this can be counteracted by giving extra oxygen by face mask, and this can be arranged if the airline is given warning in advance. In this way patients with controlled heart failure, angina, or recovered myocardial infarction (heart attack) can safely fly.

If you are in doubt the airline must be consulted in advance and the decision of its medical officer must be taken as final.

Besides the actual flight, one should also consider all the

other stresses that are part of air travel. The fear of not being on time, of forgetting something, losing the way and anxieties associated with his luggage, tickets, and customs all impose an extra mental load, often leading to an increased heart rate and subsequent exhaustion. The physical activity involved in travelling may be quite considerable, including long walks along airport corridors and climbing stairs, often whilst carrying luggage: this is tiring enough even for the seasoned traveller who is well and free from heart trouble. Much of this strain can be relieved by prior communication with the airport authorities. Careful planning will ensure that a wheeled chair is available to take you directly to the plane.

Careful consideration must be given to the choice of destination. Sudden changes in climate or altitude may be harmful. It may sound perfect in theory to take a holiday in North Africa or the Balearics, but in practice you may find yourself incapacitated by the unaccustomed heat or by not being able to sleep in strange and perhaps noisy surroundings.

Package holidays involving sight-seeing are particularly undesirable for if you are convalescing from a heart attack. The tours are often arduous, involving a great deal of walking and long and tiring coach journeys.

It must be remembered that medical services in foreign countries are not always as good as those at home and, in an emergency, adequate facilities may be lacking. In addition you may have considerable language difficulties if you have to be admitted to hospital, and the return journey home may pose great problems in these circumstances.

17

Research and the future

The last fifty years have seen the virtual elimination in the Western world of diseases such as poliomyelitis, tuberculosis, rheumatic fever, diphtheria, cerebral spinal fever, lobar pneumonia, osteomyelitis, rickets, mastoid, and many other infections. Anaesthesia has been turned from a nightmare into a pleasant experience and surgical operations made incomparably safer. All this has been made possible by the dedicated work of research doctors and scientists piecing together information gained by experiments in the laboratory and carefully trying out their results in animals and man. If ever there was a success story in man's endeavours it is in the field of medical research and the benefits it has brought to mankind.

Although coronary heart disease has not yet been conquered, there have been very substantial advances in the diagnosis and treatment not only of the illness itself but of high blood pressure, which may predispose to heart trouble.

Until the 1950s there was virtually no treatment for high blood pressure. A few doctors were aware that lowering the patient's blood sodium would lower the blood pressure and this led to treatment by a diet free of sodium and which consisted almost entirely of boiled rice and fruit. Few patients could tolerate such a monotonous diet. Today the blood sodium can be reduced by the use of diuretic medicines (water pills) and, in many patients, blood pressure can be controlled by these alone. New and more powerful medicines have been developed which are effective in controlling even the most severe cases.

Research and the future

The discovery of the 'beta blocking' drug represents a remarkable 'breakthrough' in the treatment of high blood pressure and angina. It had long been known that the control of the heart rate and blood pressure were in part under the control of chemical substances known as catecholamines which are produced at the nerve endings of the autonomic nervous system connected to the heart and blood vessels. Some years ago research workers discovered the formulae of these chemicals but their discovery had only a limited value and to a large extent remained an interesting scientific observation, with relatively little practical value in the treatment of diseases of the heart and circulation. In the 1950s research workers put forward the idea that it might be possible to develop a chemical whose formula would be so similar to that of the catecholamines that it would compete with the catecholamines and so neutralize or block their effect on the heart and circulation. Brilliant research led to the development of a series of chemical substances which would achieve the desired result and beta-blocking drugs were born. The breakthrough was achieved by building on the knowledge of physiology and chemistry established over years of patient research which at times appeared to bear no relevance to the treatment of human subjects.

The development of open heart surgery since the 1950s is another exciting and almost unbelievable advance in the treatment of heart disease that we owe to dedicated research by teams throughout the world. Until this time doctors would have considered it in the realms of impossibility to open the human heart at operation and repair damaged valves or arteries or to reconstruct the hearts of children born with holes or other cardiac defects.

Work by physiologists in animals, however, had shown that it might be possible to disconnect the heart and pass the blood through an apparatus which would substitute for the heart's pumping action and oxygenate the blood for a limited period of time. At the time this was thought to be of interest but have little relevance in the treatment of heart disease in man.

In the 1950s research was undertaken in several centres in the world to see whether this could be applied to man, and the services of doctors, physiologists, and engineers were called in to devise a 'heart–lung' machine which could be safely used in patients. Special roller pumps had to be devised with membrances to transmit the oxygen to the blood and it took several years of intensive research to produce a machine which could be tried on patients. Today the patient's heart can be disconnected from the circulation, stopped by chemical or other means, maintained by the heart–lung machine, and opened. Faults can be repaired, artificial valves inserted, or arteries replaced. Each step in such operations has been the culmination of years of research in many centres throughout the world.

Similar stories can be told about pacemakers or the whole range of medicines being introduced to control the irregularities of the heart's action in coronary heart disease. Methods of diagnosis and understanding of the mechanisms by which the heart becomes disturbed in its action have added to this success story.

Medical research can perhaps be likened to a giant jigsaw puzzle. Research workers throughout the world are putting together pieces of the puzzle but it is only when the last few pieces fall into place that the picture becomes clear and the 'breakthrough' happens. Success in research needs persistence and time; often there is disappointment and failure but the experience of the last few decades shows the tremendous strides forward that can be made in the elimination and treatment of diseases as a whole.

The future

The aim of heart research is to enable man to live his normal span of life free from heart disease. If this is not entirely possible then all means must be found at least to reduce the incidence and frequency of the disease. At the present time it would seem that some people are born with a greater likelihood of developing coronary heart disease, but there are external factors such as smoking which will increase the chances of anyone developing heart disease.

Laboratory research is being directed at finding out more about the very complex chemical and biophysical processes underlying the mechanisms of blood clotting, and the interactions of the blood with the lining of the walls of the arteries and the veins. More will have to be discovered on why the arterial walls themselves become diseased and the more precise effects that the components of the blood, including foodstuffs, hormones, other chemicals, and even viruses, may play in this process.

In the field of epidemiology, which looks at the way external influences and life-style affect populations, much has already been achieved in showing trends of the disease in various countries. However the final riddle has yet to be solved.

One thing is certain, and that is, without continuing research, we shall never make any advances in eradicating heart disease.

The research worker

Modern medical research is extremely complex and cannot be approached in the same way as if you were designing a new motor car or finding the cause of a malfunction in a television set. It is often understandably difficult for the layman to understand exactly how medical research proceeds and why more rapid progress cannot be achieved given the will, organization, and the money.

Although money is essential, it is probable that the limiting factor is the number of research workers with the drive and enthusiasm to overcome difficulties and see forward to the next step in the problem as a whole. Research workers in medicine are relatively few compared with the total population of doctors and the financial rewards and security of employment less than those of practising doctors. Often a good research worker has to be a 'rebel' and break away from the traditional thought and teaching of his elders. His mind is continually questioning and thinking out new approaches to solve a particular problem. He is for the most part an individualist and cannot be ordered to solve a particular problem but has to proceed forward in his own way. He must not be deterred by failure and indeed a 'negative' experiment often gives a lead in another direction. Often in the past his medical colleagues have had little sympathy for his endeavours and he has been labelled 'a back room boy' and made to feel inferior. Fortunately with the increasing success of medical research this attitude is now passing and the value of the research worker is becoming increasingly recognized.

It is apparent, therefore, that there is a balance between the available 'brains' for effective research and the amount of money available for their support. Too little money will hold up valuable work while an excess will be party to the law of diminishing returns. Although it could be argued that in the United States in the last decade spending on medical research has been a little excessive, this does not apply to the United Kingdom where more money is always needed to support the research endeavours which in many cases have led the world.

The support of heart research

Medical research as a whole, of which heart research is a part, is supported in the United Kingdom by three government agencies—namely, the Medical Research Council, the Department of Health and Social Security, and the universities. Each plays a valuable part in not only maintaining individual research workers but also by establishing departments within universities and special centres devoted to research. Their

Research and the future

funds have to be spread widely over a large area of research not only in heart disease but all over medical diseases as a whole and are not always adequate to obtain maximum results.

The last few decades have seen the introduction and development of the large charitable organizations entirely supported by donations from the public which are devoted to medical research. In the case of heart disease the largest of these in the United Kingdom is the British Heart Foundation. In many ways such foundations complement the government organizations in that not only do they have a greater flexibility in the use of their funds but act as an alternative source of support which can supplement that provided by the government agencies.

Similar organizations (the National Institutes for Health and the American Heart Association) support research in the United States.

As receently as the 1940s it was not thought possible that in the foreseeable future tuberculosis, poliomyelitis, cerebro-spinal fever, and many other diseases could be controlled or cured. Today perhaps we are in the same position with coronary heart disease. Let us hope that in the course of the next few years books like this one will not be needed and will be of historical interest only.

Index

Index

Index